It's Never Too Late...

The Hidden Truth About
Aging & Menopause

By

Dr. Dawn D. Andalon

Publisher: The Andalon Company, Inc. 681 Encinitas Blvd #308 Encinitas, CA 92024. While they have made every effort to verify the information here, neither the author nor the publisher assumes any responsibility for errors, omissions from or a different interpretation of the subject matter. This information may be subject to varying laws and practices in different areas, states, and countries. The reader assumes all responsibility for the use of the information.

It's Never Too Late is a work of nonfiction. Nonetheless, some names and personal characteristics of individuals or events have been changed in order to disguise identities. Any resulting resemblance to persons living or dead is entirely coincidental and unintentional.

Every effort has been made to make this book as accurate as possible. Any errors or inconsistencies are unintentional. The purpose of this book is to inform and educate. No individual should use the information in this book for self-diagnosis, treatment or as justification for accepting or declining any medical therapy for any health problem or disease. No individual is discouraged from seeking professional medical advice and treatment. This book is not supplying medical advice. Any implication of the information herein is at the reader's own risk. Any individual with a specific health problem or who is taking medication should first seek advice from his or her personal physician or healthcare provider before starting any program of self-care, especially one that includes a change in diet or levels of exercise.

The author and publisher shall in no event be held liable to any party for any damages arising directly or indirectly from any use of this material. Every effort has been made to accurately represent our products and services and its potential.

Editing by Amy Haywood
Photography by Petulapea Photography

To order this book from the author, please visit www.level4pt.com/whbooks.

NEED HELP NAVIGATING THE PHYSICAL EFFECTS OF PERI/POSTMENOPAUSE?

TALK TO THE SPECIALISTS

Schedule a complimentary consultation with one of our women's health specialists by visiting

www.level4pt.com/telephone-consultation

or

call us at (760) 503-4440

DEDICATION

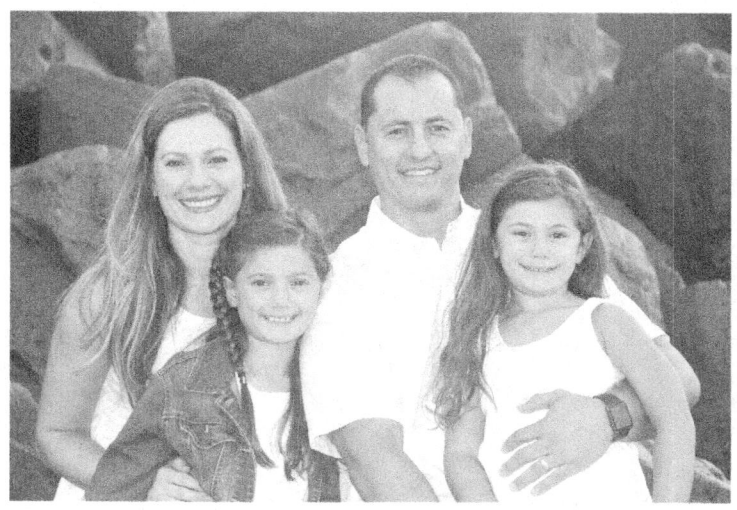

Andalon Family

Thank you to my family!

To my dear hubby- Thank you for pushing me
to be the best version of myself.

To Alexa and Sophia - For being the strong and confident girls
you are, for inspiring me to work toward my goals, and for being
one of the reasons why I continue to write books for women.
Thank you for all the laughter you bring us every day, and
I am so very proud of you both! I love you!

XOXO

CONTENTS

BEFORE YOU READ THIS BOOK, DO THIS FIRST...

Just to say thanks for reading this book, I would like to give you some special bonuses – absolutely FREE!

At the time of writing this book, thousands of people from around the world receive regular and very helpful practical health tips from the experts at LEVEL4.

Go to:
www.level4pt.com/whgifts
to download them now.

Here's what you will receive:

I'll include our *7-Minute Daily Stretching Routine Guide*, which is perfect for women aged 40 or over who wish they could move easier, bend further, stretch more...and ache much less! (value $27)

Plus two other helpful tips guides:

*7 Reasons Why Pilates Will Ease Your Pain...
and Reshape Your Life* (value $19)

10 Biggest Mistakes Women Make When Trying to Stay Fit
(value $19)

You'll be able to see them ALL instantly when you enter your name and email address at www.level4pt.com/whgifts.

TESTIMONIALS

Awesome experience! I came to Dr. Dawn to work on my core weakness & back pain and I was surprised by how much I have improved in just a few short weeks! Seriously, I went from feeling like wobbly Jell-O to feeling totally stable when doing core work like planks, push-ups, overhead squats, snatches, etc. Not only that, but Dr. Dawn corrected multiple other issues I was having as well! Knee/hip pain, low back pain...I went from having pain after every workout, to having almost none. She is crazy smart and I can't recommend her enough!!

Adriane F. – 40, Oceanside, CA

I made an appointment regarding my hip as I was researching what I could do to avoid surgery. At first I was worried it wouldn't work for me as I tried multiple practitioners in the past. I was skeptical and was unsure if this was the right path for me. I decided to give it a try and I am so thankful I did! She helped me with pain relief, and I am now able to get up and down from the floor to play with my grandkids, which is what I was so frustrated I couldn't do in the past. I learned exercises and modifications unique to my needs. I was provided exceptional care with follow-up calls to check on how I was doing. They are a talented team with a high quality of care that really wants you to succeed.

Mary S. – 58, Encinitas, CA

I would highly recommend Dr. Dawn. She is so knowledgeable and very helpful in every area. Now I am post hip surgery and attending a Pilates class. She is amazing, helping me strengthen and heal and watching that I don't push too hard. Both are very professional and friendly, and you know they genuinely care about you. Give them a try—you won't be disappointed!

Marcie F. – 71, Oceanside, CA

LEVEL4 has turned me into an addict to get in shape! They take care of you while also working your body to strengthen and tone every muscle. My friends are amazed at my transformation, and it has really helped me! I had stage 4 colon cancer and a total hip replacement, and thanks to this experience, I am more in shape than 15 years ago…and I am over 60! THEY REALLY KNOW WHAT TO DO AND WILL TAKE CARE OF YOU, TOO! They are there 100% for YOU! It is a gift I give myself, and I love working out now!

Betsy D. – 67, Rancho Santa Fe, CA

I wanted to talk about female issues! Some women are too embarrassed to discuss bladder leakage, prolapse, or overactive bladder. I've had 3 bladder sling operations and do not want a 4th. I found a very unique "all female" physical therapy clinic in Encinitas that handles all issues related to women. This clinic is unlike any other I've been to. They are training my body to be restored and healed and to strengthen my pelvic floor. I've never had so much information regarding that area. It's not just about "Kegels"; they teach the proper way and activate muscles you've never used! They are kind and comforting and you feel so informed! I highly recommend!!

Jaime C. – 45, San Diego, CA

FOREWORD

Most likely, if you've picked up this book, you are aware that something may be missing out on in your life as you are getting older. Maybe you are struggling in a body that hurts or is not performing like it once did, you are left scared, nervous, and possibly even feel hopeless. Maybe you aren't feeling like yourself and you want to feel confidence in your body again. Maybe your energy is not where you want it to be. You probably have activities that you are giving up on or pretending like it's ok if you don't continue—but you're no longer sure how to do them. You feel broken.

I know how this feels–from my own experiences and the thousands of other women I have helped.

You are confused, searching for answers.

Or, possibly, you're like some other women I know. You are ambitious and competitive, but your body feels different than it did a decade ago. You work hard every single day, and you are trying your best to stay healthy. You love challenges. You will do what it takes to achieve your best.

I know how that feels, too.

Winning at anything in life is 80 percent behavior and 20 percent head knowledge. It's not enough to *know* good health and wellness principles—it's *acting* on those principles that is important.

One of the best questions I ask clients is: "What are you missing out on in life?"

Do you like the place where you are physically? Have you lost the ability to do something you once could? If not, are you willing to own up to the fact that you are the person who is in charge of your body and your health?

You can experience success when you identify that you are ready to take action and live with more vitality and happiness so you can truly "age gracefully."

It's never too late!!

INTRODUCTION

Too many times I have heard: "I am too old for this," "My doctor said I might have to give up on this activity," or "Maybe it is just my age."

I know that is what most of us think; it is what we are led to believe after years of chatting with girlfriends, listening to mothers' or grandmothers' complaints, reading or seeing such messages in the media, or maybe clinging to an excuse that our own doctor gave us.

I am here to tell you that this kind of thinking is totally false! Who am I to give you this advice? As a physical therapist (and women's health specialist) who has worked with thousands of women over the years, I've seen women crush these myths all the time. I have witnessed some pretty amazing transformations, especially for women who are over 50 years young.

But you know what is mind-blowing? Women are constantly surrendering to the notion that "it's just the way things are," yet I've helped women continue doing the activities they love without relying on medications, surgery, or other invasive methods that the traditional medical system may recommend. The problem is that many women just don't know there IS another way. In this book you are about to read, I want to give you a new perspective. The way things have "always been done" is not the way *I* do things at my practice. Every woman deserves a chance to be heard, a chance to be seen, and a chance to discover how she can absolutely live her best life.

I grew up drawn to physical fitness. I was a gymnast and dancer, intrigued by the power of the human body. I have worked as a personal trainer, and I've gone on my own health journey and struggles with my weight, aches and pains, and motivation. I have listened to countless women state they feel like they are losing control over their body, dismissing the things they really want in life because they took the easy way out and gave up or instead got too frustrated and let go of what they once thought life would look like. From their perspective it was just easier to let it go and suffer than actually make a decision to turn it around. If they tried something new, would it even work or would they fail again?

The worst, though, is when the advice they were given was to wait it out, give up on that activity, or don't go on that vacation because they couldn't keep up or worried about how their body would limit them.

Sound familiar?

For those skeptical, nervous, or just disappointed in what you have been told by a doctor or another health professional...I hear you. If you are like me and you are listening to your gut and it tells you, "Maybe there is something better!" then do me a favor: stop and listen to that voice.

It's important to note that in addition to discussing physical changes in our "female parts," I also focus on the often neglected topics of perimenopause and postmenopause. With such little support surrounding menopause, women are frequently left wondering what else can help them cope with the physical changes they are feeling besides medications, gadgets, or the dreaded surgery. Because of my specialty in pelvic floor physical therapy, I have written specific chapters that all women need to read related to these changes that occur–information they might not hear from their doctor.

Women who are more informed about issues specific to females have greater confidence and control when it comes to their own physical health. With the lack of guidance and support on issues surrounding menopause, I thought it was important to address those first.

I'll also dive into what you can do to address chronic back pain, lack of bladder control, low libido, weight gain, or lack of energy, among other topics. Aging comes with changes to our female bodies, but I will show you that it doesn't have to limit your ability to keep up with friends and family.

Keep reading, and we will go on a journey together toward a life free from worry that your body is going to fail you and free from a life missing out on the things you love. I will show you how your life might be different with a little courage, commitment, and discipline.

CHAPTER 1

The 3 "Ps" (Peri- & Postmenopause & Your Pelvic Floor)

Menopause typically has a negative reputation in our society. While there is a sense of solidarity among us because nearly every woman experiences it, menopause is often characterized as a disease to survive rather than a natural process to experience. It can also be a difficult transition for many women given the implications for fertility or physical changes that occur.

On the other hand, some women welcome it. While everyone's journey is unique, we do have more control over our experience of menopause than we think. Specifically, the more information we have about menopause, the less of a negative effect it has on our lives! In other words, knowledge is very powerful, especially in preparation for this stage of life, but also at any point in your journey.

First, let's start with some definitions for clarity:

- *Menopause* is the point in time where a woman has not had her period for 12 months, which occurs at the average age of 51.

- **Perimenopause** is the period of two to ten years before menopause during which changes in progesterone, estrogen, and testosterone hormone levels occur.

- **Postmenopause** is the period of time after menopause.

Next, here's a brief outline of the hormonal changes that occur:

- **Progesterone** levels are the first to change, typically during the perimenopause period. This hormone contributes to sleep, calmness (anti-anxiety), and pain processing.

- **Estrogen** levels remain relatively stable until the year before the last menstrual period (the end of perimenopause). Estrogen (and estrogen variations) contributes to tissue lubrication (including the vulva), tissue elasticity (including the ligaments that help hold up your organs), heart health, sleep quality, and mood.

- **Testosterone**, on the other hand, decreases in the post menopause stage. This hormone impacts sexual desire and pleasure, energy, muscle mass, bone density, and mood.

As you can see, the perimenopause–menopause–postmenopausal life stage impacts many important areas of life, such as sleep, mental health, and weight management. Yet, pelvic health is worthy of our attention as well, as it involves basic function and deeply impacts quality of life. *Pelvic health* involves bladder, bowel, and sexual function, as well as pain-free living and moving, which often involves your *pelvic floor muscles* (or your "Kegel" muscles).

Education and information given to women is scarce for both postpartum and the menopausal stage, even though evidence has shown these periods of time in a woman's life do create more concern about pelvic floor dysfunctions. (Refer to my prior book, *Beyond Nine Months*, as I discuss postpartum physical recovery resources in more detail).

What is very interesting was a study of more than 500 women, either pregnant or postmenopausal, that discussed the disproportionate amount of information that had been provided to women during the perimenopausal stage, compared to during pregnancy (which, even so, is still lacking).[1] In fact, women were educated more in the postmenopausal stage about pelvic floor dysfunction and prevention strategies instead of during perimenopause, which is rather late; many of the common physical issues could be prevented or treated sooner. Only 34 percent of postmenopausal women received information during their peripartum period, but then 57 percent of postmenopausal women in the study expressed concern over urinary incontinence and pelvic floor dysfunctions.

Some of the common (but not normal!) pelvic health issues that occur in this stage of life include:

- *Pelvic organ prolapse*: 50 percent of women over 50 experience a change in the position of where the bladder, cervix/uterus, and/or rectum sit in the pelvis. When any of these organs sits lower down, this creates pressure, heaviness, or protrusion in the vaginal opening, or it causes difficulty with peeing or having a bowel movement. Prolapse is more common in women who had muscle tearing during childbirth, however long ago it occurred.

- *Urinary incontinence*: One in three women experiences leaking of urine with sneezing, coughing, laughing, exercising, hearing water running, or getting to the bathroom. This leaking could be anything from a dribble to full loss.

1

- *Genitourinary Syndrome*: This term describes the genital, urinary, and sexual changes related to estrogen decline. These include:

  o *Dyspareunia (pain with sex)*: One in five women experiences pain with intercourse and/or sexual activity. Pain can happen because of muscular issues, skin conditions, or vulvar/vaginal tissue dryness, irritation, or sensitivity, and can occur with initial insertion of something into the vagina, deep penetration, or after sexual activity. In addition, pain can occur either with or separately from low libido and difficulty with arousal and desire.

  o *Urethral irritation*: Includes pain in the vulvar area, pain with urination, frequent urinary tract infections, and/or an increased urgency to urinate

- *Fecal incontinence*: One in five women over 40 experiences loss of stool (from smearing on underwear to full loss) that can happen with a strong urge to go, after a bowel movement, or with activity (walking, changing positions, lifting, etc.).

- *Constipation*: When bowel movements occur less than every two to three days and/or you have the feeling of incomplete emptying, the need to strain/push, or stool that is hard, bulky, or pellet-like. Constipation often exacerbates the issues listed above due to the pressure it puts on the pelvic system.

The issues above occur due to a variety of factors, but the good news is that they can be improved and even resolved! Ultimately, perimenopausal or postmenopausal women have many health considerations. It is possible to bring joy to your experience of perimenopause or postmenopause. It's never too early, especially given recent research, and it's also never too late.

CHAPTER 2

POWER TO THE FEMALE

Are you a woman dealing with an issue you just assumed was a normal byproduct of childbirth, aging, or menopause? Maybe you had a surgery already and you are experiencing some of these confusing symptoms you didn't expect. You're not alone, and I wrote this book because so many women were telling me the same thing—"I didn't know you could fix this!"

These types of stories are what I hear on a daily basis:

Janine was diagnosed with a prolapsed bladder and feared exercising or lifting weights, which was her stress relief from a busy life with high school girls and an intense career. Her doctor told her the only way to help her symptoms was to eventually have surgery, and she was not going to stand for that being her only option.

She feared making things worse and did not want to resort to surgery.

She searched online and tried some of the exercises she read about, but she still continued to experience pressure and heaviness in the vaginal area.

We found out her real problem was that she was actually bearing down on her pelvic floor muscles instead of controlling the downward pressure on her bladder when she was standing and walking. We were QUICKLY able to diagnose and teach her how to control it by using our biofeedback device with some simple strategies and breathing exercises.

She said, "I felt this constant urge to have to go to the bathroom, and I was afraid to go on long car rides or walk with a friend by the beach. The simple things in life started to really stop me in my tracks, and I thought this is how my life was going to be now."

The good news is that Janine did not have to have surgery, but some of these stories of clients also include trauma or other emotional stress that comes with the physical issue they are experiencing. But time and time again, the commonality is the fact that a woman's life is being affected by the physical aspect of the condition, which causes even more worry and frustration. Maybe it is the area where I live (Southern California), but increasingly more information is available today that our mothers and grandmothers did not have. Some doctors are recommending a pelvic floor specialist, and also, with social media and recent press on NPR and mainstream news outlets, women are discovering more about these other resources that can help them.

Maybe you wear black yoga pants when exercising to hide the embarrassing leaking that happens with jumping jacks or fear even laughing in public because you might pee your pants. Or, maybe you were ill and your non-stop coughing made you uncontrollably leak so you had to wear a pad. Maybe just thinking about having sex again without pain seems like something in the distant past. Maybe the pressure you feel in your vaginal area when walking around is a little scary, and you're not sure if things are "in the right place" and can't remember if you ever felt that before. Maybe things feel "not quite right"—but you've just learned to deal with it for years.

Many women have never heard of a pelvic floor specialist. And many doctors, instead of referring patients to someone like me, often may prescribe a medication, suggest surgery, or, even better, tell patients to "just give it some time and see if it gets better." Well, that just isn't good enough!

A physical therapist is a musculoskeletal expert who helps people recover from an injury by using hands-on techniques like soft tissue work, joint manipulations, and exercise-based treatment to help correct faulty movement patterns and maximize their overall quality of life for the activities they want to do. While general physical therapists are not trained to address an entire muscle system called the "pelvic floor," they know about it, and would need further specialized training in how to properly assess and treat it!

Going to physical therapy school, I got two hours of lecture in my entire graduate school experience on the pelvic floor. Not to bore you with the details, but I realized after having issues, myself, that pelvic floor problems are absurdly COMMON, and there is an entire muscle system related to overcoming these embarrassing and frustrating issues. Medical doctors don't study the muscle systems as much as physical therapists do, even though they can be the source of so many medical issues like bladder leakage (called urge or stress incontinence), painful sex, prolapse (or feeling of pressure in the pelvic region), post hysterectomy issues, birth-related trauma, and many other diagnoses related to the actual muscle system of the pelvic floor.

Not only that, but back and hip pain can often be related to an undiagnosed pelvic floor issue. Some physical therapists might take weeks trying to help resolve an ongoing chronic issue that actually could be related to a deeper problem within the pelvic muscle area, which affects mobility and stability of the hips/pelvis.

It's also important to add that women who have gone through menopause will experience atrophy (or weakening) in their pelvic floor muscles, thereby affecting bladder function and increasing the risk for pelvic organ prolapse due to the drop in estrogen levels. This is also a very common symptom after a hysterectomy surgery. Many times, surgery is recommended for a prolapsed bladder (will get into this more in Chapter 8), but if women were taught the principles in this book, I believe it could lead to a lot less of these post-menopausal issues. Women 30 years ago did not have the resources we have today; pelvic floor physical therapy was extremely rare, and the activity and fitness goals of women over the age of 50 were not as popular.

Pelvic floor physical therapy can help address these issues and others by:

- Teaching proper muscle coordination and training (which only sometimes includes "Kegels" and often includes hip and core strengthening)

- Providing pertinent knowledge for optimal bladder, bowel, and sexual function

- Educating further on hormonal changes and what can be done within our profession and outside of our profession to help

- Offering fluid and food recommendations to promote better metabolism, gut, and bowel health

- Giving guidelines for exercise and movement that are safe and motivating for your current level of fitness

In addition, it is important to keep in mind that you cannot separate the pelvis from the person. The big picture considerations that make significant differences in quality of life and function during the perimenopause–menopause–postmenopausal life stage and that also impact hormone levels and muscular function either positively or negatively are: sleep quality, stress management, food intake, and regular movement. Thus, part of treatment is optimizing these areas as well. They are deeply foundational to thriving rather than surviving this stage of life because they impact everything from how you feel to your physiological processes.

It is best practice to have ALL women do a menopause check up with a pelvic floor physical therapist to be able to address issues that affect a woman's ability to stay active and happy over 50 and beyond as they age.

Gynecologists are not spending the time to address if your pelvic floor is weak, unless they tell you to do "100 Kegels a day." But that's one of the worst pieces of advice they could give!

Some of the most recent things I have heard of that were recommended by medical professionals to women are a device that you sit on to stimulate the pelvic floor muscles (YIKES), laser procedures in a medical office for tightening the vaginal wall, or a ring you place inside your vagina to help you control your bladder symptoms. The list goes on for the most ridiculous options that these medical professionals can charge for without actually recommending a specialist that helps get to the root cause of the problem!

Maybe you had a prolapse or hysterectomy surgery and the doctor says, "Just rest; it takes time," or "Everything is fine; just ease back into your old routine," without really knowing if your pelvic floor can withstand the force of jumping, walking a mile, having sex, or lifting your kids or grandkids.

Really? This type of brush-off is common, and it's not until a woman is seriously struggling with a painful issue or a seriously embarrassing one that she finally decides to seek outside help (or just stop doing the activity altogether).

Part of my purpose in becoming a pelvic floor specialist was just to get more information to women about ways they could actually help themselves without resorting to more invasive medical procedures like surgery, silly devices, procedures, or medication.

The pelvic floor and "core" are the center of your body and your powerhouse for lifting, carrying, and moving in life and recreational activities, and they cannot be ignored with aging. It is necessary to have this area functioning optimally as you age, but rarely are women given any advice that truly addresses the problem.

What is the pelvic floor, and why do I need to know this? (Trust me you need to understand this first!)

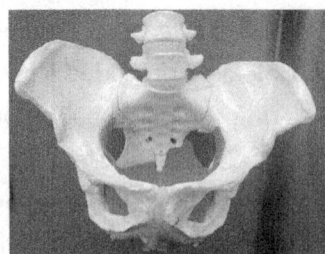 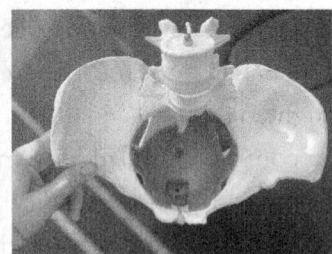

The pelvic floor can be thought of like a basket of muscles in the bottom part of your pelvis (the dark part of the picture).

These layers stretch like a hammock from the tailbone at the back, to the pubic bone in front. A woman's pelvic floor muscles support her bladder, uterus, and bowel (colon). The urine tube (front passage), the vagina, and the back passage all pass through the pelvic floor muscles. Your pelvic floor muscles help you to control your bladder and bowel; they also help sexual function.

The pelvic floor is a muscle system that should be called upon to work as much as necessary but as little as possible. It is a muscle system that is not trained like your biceps but is more like a gauge for control and stability. Subconsciously your pelvic floor needs to fire when it's called upon and is always in a state of protection and support for your pelvic organs. It's the key to bladder control—hence those embarrassing leaking moments when you sneeze or when your bladder feels full and you get a strong urge.

The "core" muscles go through significant change as they are stretched and stressed throughout your lifetime because of things like weight gain/loss, pregnancy, surgeries, trauma, etc.

The pelvic floor is the bottom portion of the "core." The diaphragm controlling your breathing is at the top, the deep abdominal muscles are in the front, and the multifidus (back stabilizing muscles) are located in the back portion. There are a ton of other muscles fully involved in controlling the movement of the middle of your body, but for the purposes of this book, I will be discussing the pelvic floor function a little bit more as I address the COMMON—but not normal—symptoms of aging. Sadly, I find that women often just live with the physical problems and fail to seek out proper treatment.

Pelvic floor issues don't always just happen because of vaginal delivery with childbirth; they can be common at any stage in life even if you did not deliver a child.

And contrary to your doctor's advice, you might NOT need Kegel exercises! They can actually create painful symptoms due to prolonged muscle holding patterns. But how would you know?

Women who have pain from a gynecological exam are often told to "just relax." But what if their muscles don't know how to relax? Yes, that is a thing. It's different with muscles like your biceps that have a voluntary ability to bend and straighten the elbow (which causes the muscle to shorten and lengthen), but your pelvic floor is on autopilot, and, at times, needs to be taught how to relax and contract properly.

When you have a pelvic floor that has difficulty with relaxation, oftentimes the symptom can be described as "pain with intercourse." Women are often feeling anxiety about being intimate with their partner and are not enjoying sex because of uncomfortable pain. Place that next to a low libido or vaginal dryness, other common symptoms of menopause, and then you have multiple issues to combat when your partner wants to be intimate. It's important for women to know it is not normal to have pain with sex, and it can be relieved with the correct treatment strategy. As with any other muscle group in the body, the pelvic floor needs proper care.

A scar from a surgery or even emotional trauma can cause an *overactive* pelvic floor. The tear may cause certain muscles to work even harder or become tight because of tension around tender spots. Some women develop an overactive pelvic floor because they try to keep their pelvic floor muscles tense for long periods.

If you have tight muscles, you may continue to feel pain if the muscles aren't treated appropriately. If you have an overactive pelvic floor, or very tight muscles, helpful treatment from a pelvic floor specialist can provide trigger point massage, or trigger point release, as it's sometimes called.

Women are not guided properly through the steps of what to do when these issues arise. Keep reading to find more specific solutions in the following chapters.

An exercise for you…

Try these two tests on yourself to see if your core and pelvic floor muscles are not living up to their potential (could mean they are the source of your problem):

a. Try doing a **jump test** for two minutes. Can you perform jumping jacks or jumping in place for two minutes straight without symptoms of joint or pelvic pain, vaginal pressure, leaking, or anything else that doesn't feel quite right? Even signs of joint pain are a red flag that should be assessed by a physical therapist.

b. The **cough test**: Place your hand over your navel while standing. Feel what happens to your abdominals when you do a fake cough. Does your stomach push out into your hand? What *should* happen is a drawing in or contraction of your "core" muscles when you cough or sneeze instead of pushing outward. This is a reflex that can be trained to have a normal functional pelvic floor and deep abdominal reaction. Your muscles should automatically tighten and draw in before a cough or sneeze, and, if they don't, you have some work to do.

Did you pass or fail?

It's not the end of the world for you if you didn't pass, but it does tell us that if you already have symptoms, then breathing, core, and pelvic floor work is going to do wonders for you!

If you had trouble with one or both of these tests, check out www.level4pt.com/womens-health to find out more.

CHAPTER 3

YOUR BLADDER DOESN'T AGE

The joy of laughter is one of life's greatest pleasures, right?

Well, not if you're a woman who can't control her bladder and suffers from urinary incontinence.

If that's you, we get it. We know it's the opposite that is true–laughing is no fun at all, and in extreme cases, the leakage that follows the simple act of laughing is so bad that you start to avoid all forms of joy.

Honestly, this is my favorite chapter. Know why? It is *the* most common misconception that incontinence is a part of aging or a side effect of childbirth. I often hear: "I will never be able to do that," OR "I just start peeing my pants, so I don't do that," OR "Ever since I had kids, I can't jump or jog." If you are a woman who is always worried about where the nearest bathroom is located when you are out in public, you have to wear a pad or Depends, or you bring an extra pair of pants when you go anywhere because you are worried about the smell if you leak, please…this is NOT something you have to live with.

In fact, a study of 290 regularly exercising women revealed a 47 percent incidence of urinary incontinence. Twenty percent stopped a routine exercise due to urinary incontinence, 18 percent modified routine exercise to avoid it, and 55 percent wore a pad during exercise...55 percent!!![2] The researchers found that jumping, running, coughing, and sneezing all promote urinary incontinence problems. This is called stress incontinence. Urge incontinence is another condition that affects many women. It is an unexpected, powerful urge to urinate that you cannot control that results in leakage before getting to the toilet.

With any type of incontinence, it seems like everything that once brought you pleasure–like sports and exercise, brunch with your girlfriends, and sex with your partner *(the things we stay alive for)*–has become your most significant source of stress and anxiety.

Let's not even talk about the terror that washes over you and drains the blood from your face before a cough or sneeze. It's enough to give you nightmares.

You live with constant fear. The fear of getting caught short. The shame of leaving a wet patch on the seat at your favorite bar or restaurant, or the traumatic shuffle back to your table trying to disguise your urine-soaked underwear and the fire-red embarrassment on your face.

Your relationship is crumbling under the stress of a lack of sex and intimacy, too. Your libido is non-existent, and your partner feels rejected, not understanding that you need to feel sexy to want sex. But wearing pads inside your lingerie or fearing the leakage caused by sexual arousal and orgasm makes you feel anything but sexy.

This stuff wasn't in your life plan, either.

You have goals, ambitions, and a desire to stay fit and healthy through exercise and staying active.

You want to walk with your girlfriends or your with your dog, hike, and swim in the ocean—to enjoy this one precious life. But it's becoming

---

2

harder and harder to live that lifestyle when you can't control your bladder.

All you want to do is stay home—close to the toilet, pads, and a change of pants. It's hard not to get down about it. You didn't think this sort of stuff happened until well into old age.

It's not something we talk about with our girlfriends. We joke and skirt around the subject, of course, but in severe incontinence cases and with any loss of bladder control, we don't want to share.

But the critical thing to remember is: *You're not alone*. It happens to all types of women. But you don't have to endure it.

Here's a clear, simple explanation for why you can't control your bladder and the range of treatments available.

What Is Urinary Incontinence?

When you cannot control your bladder and are leaking large or small amounts of urine, you probably suffer from urinary incontinence or an overactive bladder.

Women often think urinary incontinence happens because they drink too much liquid—but that's not why it's happening.

In a large proportion of cases, the problem's source has to do with your pelvic floor muscles not working properly.

However, that's not always the case, so it's important to talk to your doctor to get screened for any medical-related issues, then absolutely meet with a pelvic floor physical therapist to determine if your bladder-supporting muscles are doing their job.

Symptoms of Urinary Incontinence

When finding it hard to control your bladder, you may experience any of the following symptoms:

- Leaking urine when you laugh, sneeze, exercise, or cough.

- An unexpected, powerful urge to urinate that you cannot control that results in leakage before getting to the toilet.

- Some women may also experience spasms in the pelvic region, bedwetting, or a continuous need to go to the bathroom more than eight times in 24 hours.

Causes of Loss of Bladder Control

One of the most common causes is the lack of communication between your bladder, your pelvic floor muscles, and your brain.

The pelvic floor muscles may or may not be weak. Still, it's often the case that they are not communicating well when you get the urge to urinate, and this can become a problem over time if not resolved.

Receiving proper guidance on how to contract and relax the muscles properly—just like any other muscle in your body—is an important step to take after pregnancy, during menopause, or even at other times in a woman's life.

In some cases, the open gateway of lax pelvic floor muscles results in problems with the nerves in the bladder or urethra. Other causes can be a loss of bladder control due to extra pressure on the bladder or pelvic floor muscles because of weight gain, chronic constipation, medicines, high caffeine intake, and infection.

With the path through the urethra left open, you experience an unexpected, urgent need to urinate that results in leakage.

Women are twice as likely to suffer from urinary incontinence than men.

The strain during pregnancy, the way the pelvic floor muscles lose strength during menopause, and the shorter pathway of the female urethra make women more susceptible to an overactive bladder than men.

Types of Urinary Incontinence

There are four types of urinary incontinence that affect your ability to control your bladder, and you might find you have a combination of more than one.

1. *Stress incontinence* is a prevalent form of urinary incontinence, particularly for new moms and women going through menopause. The extra strain from pregnancy (or just from the passage of time) on the bladder and urethra causes weakened pelvic floor muscles. This, in turn, causes urine to escape during actions like laughter, exercise, or sneezing.

2. *Urge incontinence* is most often experienced by older women. It involves feeling an unexpected, powerful need to pee after drinking a glass of water, hearing running water, while sleeping, and more. In most cases, nothing much comes out when you use the toilet. You might leak before you get to the toilet, or it may be a feeling you experience more than eight times in 24 hours.

3. *Total incontinence* is when your bladder is unable to retain any urine for any length of time.

4. *Overflow incontinence* occurs when your bladder never fully empties, so trickles of urine leak out continuously or once you have finished urinating.

How to Treat Loss of Bladder Control

In many cases, the treatments for urinary incontinence are surprisingly simple—but don't try to self-diagnose. The diagnosis part is complex. Urinary incontinence is usually an outcome of a problem somewhere else in the body, and it's not directly associated with the bladder. The many different types of urinary incontinence each have their own specific treatments.

Bladder Control Treatments

Some of the most prevalent urinary incontinence treatments include retraining your pelvic floor muscles and keeping track of your bladder habits–those that are both dysfunctional and those that are healthy.

It is possible to improve the function of pelvic floor muscles by doing specific pelvic floor exercises and breathing techniques to retrain them. It isn't always about strengthening the muscles; instead, it's about strengthening the sequencing and connection to the system that can control the muscles—aka "get your brain to connect to your body." This connection is often lost with hormonal changes, trauma, pregnancy, or labor/delivery, and surgeries and it could be the missing link for you. It's not enough to "just do the exercises" that a doctor may suggest; what's really needed is the expertise of a professional who knows how to get the muscles to work and fire properly! Your brain has a lot to do with bladder control and reactions. Many times the pathway from the brain to your pelvic floor muscles or bladder could be confused or interrupted. Sometimes it may require slowing down your breathing and teaching the muscles how to sync with your brain; in this way, we effectively reset that pathway from the brain to the muscles.

Many times, it is not just about strengthening where we need to focus, and that is why you could be doing Kegels yet the symptoms never improve. It just needs the right type of training program. Or, if this is truly a weakness issue and your pelvic floor muscles can't sustain the graded contraction when an impact or increased force is placed upon them, then strengthening in the right manner and progression can be hugely successful.

Here is an exercise you can do on your own to train your pelvic floor for the stress placed on it:

> Think of squeezing a blueberry in your vaginal opening, and keep it there. While you hold it, try doing a fake cough. After the cough, release the imaginary blueberry. Repeat ten times; perform at least three to four times per day. This is training a reflex that normally should work to contract your pelvic floor before a sneeze or cough. Sometimes your pelvic floor is doing the opposite and pushing those muscles out, rather than "in and up," with a physically demanding effort or during a cough or sneeze. Try performing this action prior to lifting something heavy or lifting an object from the floor. It's like a "pre- set" contraction of your pelvic floor *before* you exert yourself.

Along with retraining your pelvic floor muscles to improve bladder control, it's also helpful to keep track of your dysfunctional bladder habits as well as recognize the healthy habits you already have.

First, it's important to keep track of any DYSFUNCTIONAL BLADDER HABITS you might have. Any of the following habits could lead to a long-term issue:

1. *"Just in case" peeing.* You are anticipating that long car ride, you see the fitness routine that you are planning to do, or you see a bathroom prior to getting on an airplane and decide, "I should just go now before I really have to." Repetitive "just in case" peeing leads to dysfunctional habits and a programmed response for the bladder to empty even before it's full. This can lead to more urgency in the long run.

2. *Semi-squatting on the toilet.* In this case, please sit your entire bottom on the toilet. I don't care what you have to do to clean the toilet seat (wipe off the seat, use extra toilet paper on the seat, etc.), but if you semi-squat over the seat, you aren't fully emptying your bladder because your pelvic floor muscles can't completely relax.

3. *Don't strain to pee.* Pushing or forcing out urine also does not come from a place of full relaxation of the pelvic floor.

4. *Don't do your Kegel exercises on the toilet.* This will confuse your bladder and muscles. I use this as a cue to know which muscles you actually need to contract during a Kegel exercise, but please don't do it while sitting on the toilet; save it for other times during the day.

Now, see what you are doing that is on the list for HEALTHY BLADDER HABITS:

1. *Sit all the way down on a toilet when you go to the bathroom.* Sitting all the way down will allow your bladder to empty completely.

2. *Urinate every three to four hours* on average.

3. *Aim for an "8 Mississippi" count* as a normal amount of time you should be actually peeing. If you are going a lot longer than that, then you are probably waiting too long to void. On the other hand, if it is markedly less time than that, then you are going too often and you have a high level of urgency. This could mean you need to do some bladder training, and try to see if you can train yourself to hold it an extra 15 to 20 minutes each time you get the urge.

4. *You are able to hold the need to urinate during the night and not wake up to pee.* This habit is common, especially after pregnancy and post-menopause, but fairly easy to train. Many times, this will be what

we see on a voiding log (see example/diagram). Also, when you are getting really great sleep, you won't activate the sensation in your brain that gives you the urge to get up at night.

5. *Positioning when urinating.* Keep a slight forward tilt in the pelvis with a straight spine. Don't curl your tailbone underneath you as this places more pressure on the pelvic organs and doesn't allow for full relaxation of the pelvic floor muscles.

6. *Avoid constipation.* Eating fiber in your diet, staying hydrated, and keeping ahead of any constipation symptoms can prevent you from overstraining and having extra pressure on your pelvic floor, which can even impact bladder function.

7. *Go before or right after sex.* Urinary tract infections are unquestionably associated with sexual intercourse. Cystitis is common after sexual intercourse and is another word for inflammation of the bladder. One of the major reasons that intercourse is thought to be associated with urinary tract infections is that penetration can put pressure on the urethra. This can irritate the urethra or force bacteria up into the urethra and toward the bladder. In turn, this raises the likelihood of infection.

Other things to try on your own first for any type of incontinence:

1. *Diaphragmatic breathing exercises:* practice in sitting, standing, and walking. (See "Diaphragmatic breathing" on our LEVEL4 PT & Wellness YouTube channel for instruction).
2. *Yoga poses* to promote opening of the hips and to stretch the inner thighs or a pigeon stretch can also be very helpful to release increased tension in the pelvic floor muscles. This will help your muscles to activate more efficiently.
3. *Bladder training:* Train your bladder to retain higher volumes of urine by scheduling your trips to the bathroom. Write down how

often you go to the toilet over a series of days. Next, create a 24-hour timetable for your bathroom visits with an extra 15-minute break between each trip. (see voiding log pictured)

LEVEL4
PT & Wellness

24 Hour Voiding Log

Name:_____   Date:_____

Time of Day	Type & Amount of Food & Fluid Intake	Amount Voided Ounces, S / M / L, or Seconds	Amount of Leakage S, M, L	Was Urge Present 1,2,3	Activity With Leakage
Midnight					
1:00 AM					
2:00 AM					
3:00 AM					
4:00 AM					
5:00 AM					
6:00 AM					
7:00 AM					
8:00 AM					
9:00 AM					
10:00 AM					
11:00 AM					
NOON					
1:00 PM					
2:00 PM					
3:00 PM					
4:00 PM					
5:00 PM					
6:00 PM					
7:00 PM					
8:00 PM					
9:00 PM					
10:00 PM					
11:00 PM					

Comments: _____

_____

Number of pads used today: _____

Filling out this log helps you to see your daily habits, and it is a practical tool I use in my office to train new habits. You can learn a lot from documenting your daily intake of fluids, food, and how many times you go to the bathroom in a day.

4. *Diet changes*: Other irritants that you consume on a daily basis could be making your symptoms worse. Try drinking less caffeine and cutting out fizzy drinks, citrus, acidic foods, alcohol, and smoking to see a decrease in symptoms.

If you have diligently tried all of the above consistently for at least 30 days and your symptoms have not resolved, then *the #1 most effective treatment for urinary stress incontinence and a loss of bladder control is to see a specialist, called a pelvic floor physical therapist, who treats this condition.*

Finding the root cause of your bladder control problems—to treat it and stop it from returning—is key. Kegels and bladder training might be only part of the solution., but they aren't the total solution, and they're unlikely to work in isolation to fix your problems.

Cynthia, a former client, was able to find relief when specialists identified the root cause of her incontinence:

Cynthia's granddaughter had begged her to play on a trampoline with her, but when she began jumping, she started to lose her bladder control. It was enough to make her believe that she was "too old" to jump anymore because she couldn't control herself.

Her friend laughed with her saying the same thing happens to her, so she doesn't even try it. It wasn't until later when I met Cynthia at an event and gave a talk on pelvic floor and bladder control, that her ears perked up. She admitted to me later how embarrassed she was, and she wondered if she could solve it.

Cynthia's story is incredibly common. In fact, this is usually the top women's health issue that women do *not* seek help for because they do not know someone can actually help them resolve it. Doctors and women often discount incontinence as being a normal part of aging or motherhood. Doctors will direct women to do Kegel exercises without any sort of follow up or direction; and other women will often say amongst each other that it "just happens after you have babies or when you get older; join the club." I hear it in the women's restroom at the gym; I hear it when women are socializing; and I hear it from my friends. It can actually be simpler to resolve than you think because this is a reflex that can be trained along with pelvic floor muscle control.

So, what do pelvic floor specialists actually do to help you?

A pelvic floor specialist will guide you with a possible need for some internal massage work to release those tight muscles so you can generate a stronger contraction. Trust me, it is not as invasive as going to see your gyno! They can also teach you how to do the appropriate exercises for the exact problem you are having (and explain why!) to help you progress toward the activities that tend to activate your symptoms. As your pelvic floor learns what it is supposed to do, the specialist will integrate your pelvic floor-specific exercises with activities that are part of your daily routine or exercise.

After the specialist gets a baseline to see what your muscles can do well and what they can't do in static positions, then she gradually increases the intensity with functional movements like squats and low-impact jumping jacks, which can be an excellent and successful way to train your body in the way it is meant to function.

Urge incontinence may be treated a little bit differently, involving some of the above strategies, plus getting a baseline of what your pelvic floor and core system are capable of. Then the specialist can use tricks with your brain and some bladder training. Try any of the following strategies the next time you get a strong urge that seems like it is difficult to control:

1. Count backward from ten when you get the urge to pee to see if it goes away.

2. Take some slow deep breaths when you get the urge to go, and see if that helps you to control it.

3. Think of engaging your pelvic floor muscles to stop the urge. Wait five to ten seconds and repeat number one and two to see if the urge is still present.

Bottom line: Incontinence is not going to fix itself, and you need some professional guidance. The muscles that help support your bladder and other pelvic organs have to be taught the right way to function as your hormones cause those tissues to change during menopause. The good news is that you really don't just have to live with it!

For more incontinence tips like this, please visit this special information website: www.level4pt.com/stress-incontinence. You'll find *A Women's Guide to Improve Symptoms of Stress Incontinence*, a free 15-page guide, waiting for you that shows you six more amazing tips to stop the embarrassment of "leaking" with sneezing or exercise!

The next few sections relate to issues for women of all ages, so read on, ladies!

CHAPTER 4

BACK PAIN

- -

Dr. Andalon, my name is Casey. I'm 51, and I was recently diagnosed by my primary doctor with having L4-L5 and L5-S1 bulging discs following an MRI scan. I've now suffer with chronic back pain, stiffness, and, at times, severely painful sciatica symptoms for nine months.

At first the bulging disc symptoms were very mild. They have gradually become more painful to the point that they are interfering with my life.

I've seen numerous physicians, chiropractors, acupuncturists, and massage therapists— with no relief. I feel the problem just continues to get worse! My doctor referred me to a spine surgeon who, of course, recommends surgery since nothing else has worked.

Do you have any advice for someone like me? Is there a specific exercise for a bulging disc I can perform?

I'm just incredibly stiff when I wake up in the morning, I'm having difficulty sitting at work, and I feel it throughout the day, which means I can't do things as easily as I'd like. Any advice?

As a busy woman, Casey was frustrated by the aches and pains in her back that were slowing her down. Lifting grandkids, a heavy laundry basket, or putting Christmas decorations away can all put extra strain on the back. If you can identify with Casey, and it's been months (or even years!) where you haven't felt your best due to chronic back pain, then read on.

Back pain in women over 40 and beyond has many causes, but three of the main causes are posture changes, repetitive strain, and loss of muscle tone due to hormonal changes.

Our habits in life affect posture, and if you have spent years sitting at a desk hunched over with repetitive activities at your job, or had to lift boxes or perform any type of manual labor, usually by the time you hit the 40s and 50s your body starts reminding you it can't recover quite like it used to. Those normal aches and pains, feeling stiff and achy when you get out of bed, etc., start becoming a daily occurrence as your body begins to respond and not react as quickly as it once did. These postural stresses over time can lead to acute or chronic back pain if you aren't careful to do daily maintenance work to keep the stress and pain from coming back. Many times our joints become stiff from holding one position for long periods of time; the muscles adapt to this position, and the stiffness and soreness need more attention.

If you have not already experienced back pain in your first 40 to 50 years of life, you are one of the few. But for many women, the changes in hormone, muscle loss, and bone density can exacerbate painful back symptoms occurring later in life. As a result, you will need more muscle stability, strength, and control, especially in your pelvis and back, in order to take the stress off the joints.

What about the changes in your spine? Without proper muscle support and the ability to recruit strength from your core during these tasks, your spine will take the brunt of the burden, which is what causes the back pain.

If you sound like Casey, the great news is that I have plenty of tips and advice to help reduce those bulging disc symptoms and improve your life.

But first, other common complaints we hear in the clinic from clients who have been diagnosed with a bulging disc or a muscle strain are with activities such as:

- Bending forward or backward
- Sitting
- Twisting
- Lifting
- Carrying
- Exercising/sporting activities (lifting weights, weightlifting, etc.)
- Going from sitting to standing
- Sleeping

Lumbar bulging discs can also result in **weakness, numbness, and tingling in the legs, as well as muscle spasms**.

Bulging disc symptoms can worsen with coughing, sneezing, and bending.

When a lumbar bulging disc exerts pressure on the sciatic nerve, the resulting symptoms are commonly referred to as sciatica (see Chapter 6 for more specific information on sciatica).

Understanding and treating L4-L5 and L5-S1 disc bulges in your spine when you first begin to feel pain can prevent costly medical treatments and prevent surgery.

It is important to understand why your lower back hurts or why you are experiencing symptoms.

Unfortunately, rather than seek the advice of a professional, many confuse the situation by trying to self-diagnose via internet "research" or by taking the advice of well-meaning yet ill-advised friends. Without the guidance of a specialist, most people end up doing the wrong thing and resort to spine surgery without ever getting to the root cause. In the long term, this can lead to multiple surgeries and a gradual loss of mobility and independence.

A recent study demonstrated that early surgery in patients with 6 to 12 weeks of radicular pain leads to faster pain relief when compared with prolonged conservative treatment, but the long-term outcome may not be the most advantageous one.[3] Researchers found that in the early surgery group the initial pain returned one to two years after surgery with seemingly no improvement of symptoms. Therefore, the conservative route proved to be worth it in the long run.

If you decide to take the conservative approach, the first thing you need to do is find the exact cause for your disc bulges, which have now caused you lower back or sciatica pain. Finding the source and the cause of your pain will help you identify the correct treatment and prevent further damage that can cause lifelong pain.

You might have days where you wake up feeling good with only minor disc bulge symptoms in your low back, leg, buttock, calf, or foot. But then by the time you commute to work and sit at your desk, you feel it somewhat irritated—but you don't need painkillers just yet. By mid-morning or halfway through the day you start to feel some serious pain. And, as has become routine, you take your painkillers in preparation for the looming severe pain (I'm guessing you know what the pain is like).

By the end of the day, even after the second dose of medication, you're in horrible pain again, dreading the endless drive back home.

In reality, you can't wait to get home to cry.

When that doesn't work, you then frantically search for a resolution on your own via YouTube or Google. You probably ask friends, coworkers, or family members if they have had similar experiences and what they did

---

3

about it. And when their advice fails, you then decide to try other remedies that promise the relief you're so desperately seeking; these can include epidural injections, chiropractic adjustments, acupuncture, and massages, to name a few.

When they, too, fail to deliver the results you were promised, you quickly realize it was only a false sense of hope. You feel like you have nowhere else to turn, and you just have to deal with it for the rest of your life.

But it doesn't end there. After weeks and even months have gone by, nothing has helped, so you return to your primary doctor (for at least the third or sixth time) where you hear the dreaded words: *"I'm going to refer you to the spine specialists."*

Sound familiar?

Using surgery as a way to treat bulging disc symptoms is a common mistake, especially if the root of the problem has not been assessed.

Will it go away by itself?

Contrary to popular thinking, the pain won't go away on its own.

FACT: Back pain will never completely go away unless you change something.

How to Defeat This Frustrating Problem That Hinders You from Staying Active

Some solutions you can implement today to alleviate back pain are to:

Avoid sitting for longer than 20 minutes.

The most common cause of lower back pain is postural stress. Up to 90 percent more pressure is put on your back when you sit versus when you stand. One reason is that, if you're like most Americans, you habitually sit in ways that cause tension and imbalance in your back and neck. This applies to sitting at work, in the car, and at home.

So many of us are guilty of the same common mistakes that increase postural stress and ultimately cause back pain. Over our lifetime, subconscious habits form and make it easy for us to miss when we're putting additional stresses on our bodies. This is the main reason why health professionals now consider sitting to be the "new smoking" and why it's taking literally years off your life.

Humans weren't designed to sit for long periods of time. The body is a perpetual motion machine. When you're sedentary, your muscles get less oxygen and nutrients from your blood. The rule of thumb is to frequently change postural positions and take movement micro-breaks for every 20 minutes of sitting throughout the work day. Another helpful strategy is to drink lots of water because it keeps you hydrated, which is healthy, and it forces you to get up and move in order to use the bathroom!

If you sit for more than 20 minutes, you're stressing your core muscles significantly more than they can cope. If you haven't done anything to retrain them then you're adding to your own back pain problem. If you are sitting at a computer for any length of time, try placing a pillow or cushion in the small of your back for maximum comfort and support. This is a great temporary fix, but retraining and continuing to do exercises for your core muscle group will allow you to sit comfortably for more than 20 minutes.

Set your desk to the proper height (think of your elbows at a 90-degree angle when you are working at a computer).

If you sit at a desk all day, this is a huge contributor to back pain. When you set the desk below elbow height, you're only adding to your troubles and prolonging ill health. At elbow height, you constantly must lean forward, which is, without a doubt, the worst position for maintaining a healthy spine and reducing the occurrence of back or neck pain. No other position adds more stress to your spine than standing (or walking) while leaning forward. You might be tempted, for example, to use the grocery cart if you are walking through the store as support, but this will only help for the first few minutes.

Work on flexibility…check out the stretches in the BONUS section of this book.

Flexibility exercises are very important. Many people get their activity through long walks, playing sports, and going to the gym. Yet, how many people actually put time aside to increase their flexibility—or even associate this with exercise? Flexibility exercises always seem to be overlooked, but they really shouldn't be. Stretches before and after exercise can help, however, their main focus is to get rid of the lactic acid that built up during exercise. What you avoid doing in your daily routine can have a big impact on your back pain.

So please, begin to implement flexibility exercises as part of your daily routine today!

Take frequent "movement breaks."

Minimizing your time sitting throughout the day will help keep your spine healthy. And if the core muscles are not working like they should, you're likely to suffer long-term problems. Being weak compromises both the structural support and upright posture of the body. Therefore, it is important to release tension in the back as well as to build strength.

MY TOP 6 FAVORITE Exercises for "Desk Break Time" to perform daily:

1. *Diaphragmatic breathing:* (more detailed above) Position yourself on your back with knees bent; keep the shoulders and neck relaxed. Inhale through the nose and exhale through the mouth, allowing

the rib cage to expand side to side and the belly to rise. Imagine the air flowing all the way down into your pelvis as you inhale and the ribs expand like an umbrella opening and closing. Repeat for one to two minutes focusing on the breath going into your torso and all the way down below your navel. This is a key part of Pilates exercises, which we will discuss more in the next chapter.

2. *Pelvic floor activation with breathing:* Next, add the breathing with the pelvic floor activation by inhaling as in the first exercise, keeping the body relaxed. Upon exhale, imagine yourself stopping the flow of urine and stopping yourself from passing gas by bringing the urethra and the anus together on the exhale. Another cue that has worked well in my practice is imagining holding a blueberry in your vaginal area and lifting that blueberry up on your exhale only. So, you stay relaxed on the inhale and exhale with the pelvic floor muscle lift. Repeat 10 to 15 times, five times a day in this position, then in standing or sitting. DO NOT PERFORM pelvic floor exercises while sitting on the toilet; this will confuse your muscles and interrupt healthy bladder habits!

3. *Bridging with pelvic floor activation:* This exercise will be just like #2, but on your exhale and pelvic floor contraction, you will lift your hips up like a bridge exercise while adding a gluteal (butt) squeeze. Engage the pelvic floor and glutes on the exhale, and inhale as you lower your hips. Repeat 10 to 15 times, three sets.

4. *Squats with breath work:* Here is one of my favorites because it encourages a functional movement you do throughout the day anyway! Perform in front of a chair or a box by standing on the exhale, and inhale as you sit back down. You will engage your pelvic floor, glutes, and lower abdominals upon standing and during the exhale. To coordinate this exercise may take a few days, but keep practicing to train your brain to connect to the pelvic floor and core muscles again!

5. *Wall angels for posture:* This one I added to the list to reverse the rounded shoulders and forward head posture women spend so much time in over their lives. Plus, it also helps if you find yourself at a computer or hunched over a desk for long hours. For this exercise, keep your upper back against the wall and step out with your feet. The upper back stays in contact with the wall, and arms will be out at a 90-degree angle from the shoulders. Maintain elbows and forearms against the wall while sliding your arms up and down as if making a snow angel. (Yes, I grew up in Ohio in the snow!) Repeat ten times sliding up and down, feeling the shoulder blades moving and upper back muscles engaging. If you can't maintain your arms against the wall, or this hurts your shoulders, then you probably have really tight chest and shoulder muscles, so modify this exercise by keeping at least your elbows against the wall. (You may need to see a physical therapist if you are having shoulder or neck pain and you are that tight!)

6. *Deadlifts with a broomstick on your back:* You are doing this already all day when you bend to pick up something from the floor, but many times you are using the wrong muscles. You need to incorporate proper breathing and engage the right muscles in these lifting mechanics so you keep your back and pelvic floor healthy. Inhale, but don't fully let go of your muscles as you lower. This is more of a hip exercise and a healthy one for your back if you are doing it correctly. Your back should not round! Repeat ten times, perform three sets, and don't forget to breathe!

The purpose of these exercises is to start integrating your breathing with your pelvic floor in order to encourage healthy habits when caring for grandchildren, performing tasks around the house, and doing all the active things you do in life! Use these as "go-to" exercises throughout your life.

Finally, see a physical therapist that specializes in back pain!

Easily, the fastest way to settle back pain is to have an expert help you. Most of the time, and on their own, exercises just aren't enough to unlock the problem.

If you have joints that have become locked, stiff, or stuck, there is only one way for them to become loose—and that's by hand. (No, I am not talking about going to a chiropractor!)

The muscles and joints that surround your lower back, pelvic girdle, groin, and hip area will now be very tight and tense. So, manual therapy techniques with massage and joint mobilizations done by a physical therapist are required to relax them. These joints will likely be much easier to unlock with the right techniques. When the joints are unlocked, you will feel much freer, looser, more relaxed, and much more like your former active self, especially when followed up by the right types of strengthening exercises.

The techniques that a specialized physical therapist will use prepare the body to work out and exercise, meaning you are going to be much safer, have more movement, feel stronger, and get your energy back faster. Also note, sometimes women who have diastasis recti (abdominal separation) after pregnancy that never healed, had an abdominal surgery or hysterectomy in the past, or had excessive weight gain around the abdominal area can sometimes see an increase in lower back pain symptoms. A women's health physical therapist is specially trained on how to treat this—and even more effectively than a general physical therapist.

For more back pain tips, please visit this special information website: www.level4pt.com/back-pain. You'll find a free 17-page tips guide waiting for you that shares more ways to finally get some relief.

CHAPTER 5

GETTING STRONG FROM THE INSIDE OUT WITH PILATES

This is a perfect segue from the last chapter. If you're suffering from back, groin, or pelvic pain, you need to get the core group of muscles working properly; otherwise, it is very unlikely that you will begin to feel great as you get older.

The best way to protect your back is to activate your pelvic floor and transverse abdominis (those deep abdominals) with targeted exercises like bridges, pelvic tilts, and other core activation exercises like I had mentioned previously, not just crunches and planks. This is the one single thing that can help women of all ages.

Pilates is the hidden secret for back pain relief

Pilates has been shown to help with back pain relief, especially with targeted exercises. While many other forms of physical activity can magnify body pain, Pilates is a great choice for those currently suffering or those wishing to avoid pain risk. Pilates also offers a path to burning calories and losing weight that, otherwise, would not be accessible to those suffering from back pain.

Customized Pilates exercise tailored to your weaknesses can be a missing link in combatting the effects of changes in muscle tone and bone density due to aging. It also is helpful for women who have joint-related pain or arthritic changes.

For years now, people ranging from health experts to celebrities have touted the benefits of Pilates, singing the praises of how the regimen sculpts the body without the bulk of weightlifting.

But there are many other advantages of Pilates beyond just developing that toned body.

A big part of my training and my practice now focuses on Pilates and using the principles of Pilates to encourage healthy posture with stability and mobility of the spine, especially for women over 50.

Pilates instruction can vary from place to place depending on the instructor's training and style, but when taught by a rehab professional, it maximizes using the deep core muscles of the "powerhouse"—the abdominals, back, and pelvic floor—to support your posture and learn how it all integrates together to improve your performance in life (and your symptoms, if that is the case).

The exercises and instruction serve the purpose of allowing the shoulders to relax, the neck and head to move freely, and of relieving stress on the hips, legs, and feet, all while using your pelvic floor and abdominals in sync with your breathing.

Pilates is three-dimensional, working the entire body. It is an overall body fitness system that addresses imbalances, core control, strength, flexibility, movement efficiency, and balance. It is low-impact, and it works multiple muscle groups at the same time.

Pilates exercise is commonly thought to strengthen the core muscles. Why is that important? Your spine stability and trunk control are an integral part of spinal function. It takes a lot of stress off the joints in your spine. In the lower back, the deep spinal muscles span the space between the twelfth rib and the pelvis. They help to stabilize and mobilize the lower back. These muscles also protect the abdominal organs, control forward bending, and assist in backward and side bending of your spine.

They also help support and maintain the normal spinal curve in the lower back, giving the spinal column its resiliency and capacity to absorb shock as it connects the pelvis and chest in alignment on the vertical axis. If the deep spinal muscles of the lower back are too tight, the lower back is too rigid to allow a normal range of movement.

Being weak compromises both the structural support and upright posture of the body. Therefore, it is important to release tension in the back as well as to build strength.

As I noted in Chapter 4, taking frequent "movement breaks" and minimizing your time sitting throughout the day will help keep your spine healthy. Flexibility exercises are also very important, and they are part of a good Pilates program. If you are someone who is noticing stiffness more frequently after exercise *and* stretching, then you will really benefit from a Pilates routine.

Alignment and posture are KEY elements for improving even the appearance of your abdominals and relieving back pain. Creating a position to decrease the pressure in the intra-abdominal area is essential. You can firm up the midline of your abs, and, when instructed properly, you can help alleviate symptoms from other pressure-related problems (such as pelvic organ prolapse, hernia, varicose veins, and hemorrhoids) without tackling the root cause.

Here are some principles of the Pilates method and steps you can take on your own to begin making some changes:

1. *Create length in the spine (get "taller").*

If you do yoga, you've probably heard this one before. It's a fantastic cue.

Imagine that you are adding space in between the vertebrae. Start at the bottom of the spine, and gently make your way up the spine, feeling that you're getting taller and taller until you make it all the way to the crown of the head. This simple action may very well already make you feel lighter and more confident, and things may even seem a little less "heavy"—a morale-booster! *(When our posture is slouchy, this actually weighs down onto the muscles of the spine as well as the organs in the torso, thus making you feel heavier!)*

2. *Employ "elevator" breathing.*

Once you've found length in your body, add the breath. This breathing exercise will help to bring the breath down into the belly so it can fill the entire body.

Start the inhale breath in your belly; then let it travel up the torso like an elevator, filling the rib cage, sides of the body, and finally the lungs. Exhale; come back down the "elevator," emptying the lungs, ribs, and belly.

Inhale: belly, rib cage, pelvic, and lungs fill up
Exhale: pelvis, lungs, rib cage, belly empty out

This is an excellent breathing tool when you are experiencing any pain in your body as well.

3. *Open your chest.*

Roll the shoulders a few times, front to back; then do one last shoulder roll, forward, and up and back. From there, very gently and lightly, let the shoulders release and drop themselves onto the rib cage, as naturally as you can. Your shoulders should feel more open or wider.

Keep this opening action in the shoulders, and bring your breath into the space between the shoulder blades. A simple way to perform this exercise is to visualize sticking your chest out just a bit.

Avoid squeezing the shoulder blades together. This helps remove stress in the shoulder area. Still think of softening the front ribs downward to avoid pressing the rib cage out (or flaring the ribs), especially if you want to improve diastasis recti.

4. *Now use the abdominals and pelvic floor the right way!*

Activating the pelvic floor and deep abdominal muscles will sustain and support the length in the spine that we are aiming for, and this is essential for healing any pelvic floor or back issues.

In regard to bettering our posture, engaging the pelvic floor will help to sustain the core musculature at the base of the torso.

You may notice that adding Kegels to your walk helps to generate an "uplifted" feeling to your body while continuing to tone the lower body. To sustain good posture, a healthy and toned pelvic floor is essential.

Remember, your breath should remain steady, and *incorporating movement* to any Kegel work will help to integrate the pelvic floor exercises into the overall functionality of the body by creating connections and strengthening deep core muscles; this is what we're aiming for!

In Pilates, we teach women to integrate the pelvic floor (i.e., do Kegel first, and then pull the belly button in with your EXHALE).

Think of it this way:

1. Slightly close and "lift" the pelvic floor (think of holding a blueberry in at your vaginal area and keep it lifted).

2. Pull the area below your belly button toward the spine very slightly; imagine the tips of the hips moving toward each other.

This will activate the transverse abdominal and core musculature, creating a kind of corset of support around the spine. It's a lovely way to feel supported, uplifted, and even a bit "lighter."

5. *Position your rib cage right over your pelvis.*

Bring your attention to the rib cage, which often will be positioned in front of the hips (almost like your ribs are flaring out), imagining that you want to align vertically the back of the head with the back of the pelvis.

The pull on your abdominals might feel greater when your rib cage is not aligned right over your hips. Think of growing taller and keeping those ribs right over your hips in standing or sitting, which creates less tension in the abdominal area, allowing you to breathe more freely. The position of your ribs *does* make a difference.

6. *Release a deep breath (or give a big "sigh").*

Sighing releases tension and invites us to breathe deeply. A full breath oxygenates the body, nourishing and helping to strengthen the postural muscles surrounding the spine.

It's also a great way to release tension in the body and mind.

7. *Relax what doesn't need to be "working."*

You might also recognize this cue from yoga classes; it is another wonderful tip for good posture and also for finding focus and relieving stress in day-to-day life. How does this look in daily life?

You know how sometimes when you're working hard on something, you realize at one point that you're tensing up other parts of the body, say the forehead, jaw, or shoulders, as if these parts of the body want to "work" with you? Bring your attention to the feet and legs; although you're maintaining tone there, can the toes, for example, relax a bit more? Or maybe the hips?

Then see if the shoulders and jaw are relaxed. And, finally, relax the facial muscles. Bring your gaze a bit further ahead of you, and think of relaxing all the "skin" of your face. This helps to calm and focus the mind by bringing the attention back to the present moment. And remember to keep breathing (we're about to cover why breathing is so important)!

By aiming to keep the spine long and the body properly aligned, you can most definitely feel the effects on the mind, possibly bringing on a more positive, confident, and aware mind and body to support the center of your body and improve the appearance of your abdominals!

Proper Breathing Can Ease Back Pain and Improve Pelvic Floor Function

Breathing is the most underrated exercise we take for granted, but it is sometimes the most healing. It is the foundation of training for women— no matter where you are in life—and, most importantly, it will help you regain mobility, decrease pain, increase blood flow and circulation to promote healing, and decrease stress and anxiety.

Whether your struggle is with back pain, recovering from a hysterectomy, experiencing pelvic pain, or dealing with incontinence issues, breathing is the best place to start for rehabilitating and resetting your body.

Proper breathing is incredibly important for healthy pelvic floor function. Our primary breathing muscle is the diaphragm, a dome-shaped muscle that operates like a parachute. It connects to the lower part of the ribcage. The intercostals, little muscles that fit between your ribs, also play a primary role in breathing.

These secondary breathing muscles, known as scalenes, are located in front of the neck, the pectoralis in the chest, the muscles from behind the ear that connect to the sternum, and the upper trapezius (top of shoulders).

Let's take another look at the diaphragm. When we bring in air from the mouth or nose, the lungs expand and the diaphragm muscle moves down toward the pelvic floor. So, on the inhalation, the diaphragm pushes our organs down into a sack called the peritoneum. And where does that sack of muscles get pushed? To the pelvic floor.

This is why breath is such an important part of pelvic floor work. When we breathe in, the pelvic floor is receiving the breath and the downward-moving organs. As we exhale, the breath goes up and out. The organs also move up. A healthy pelvic floor stretches as we breathe in *and* contracts slightly as the breath goes up and out. This is a subconscious process.

Connecting it all together

We've looked at the connection between the diaphragm and the pelvic floor, but there's another key player in the healthy function of the pelvic floor: our abdominals.

The transverse abdominis, the deepest abdominal muscle, is like a corset that goes all the way around the lower torso, attaching at the bottom ribs. The fibers of the transverse abdominis are horizontal, which means when they're contracted, they pull in the diameter of the abdomen (imagine tightening a belt). These muscles also serve a purpose in exhaling the breath.

If you have "poor" posture or spend a lot of time sitting in chairs, your transverse abdominis muscle will be weak. This, in turn, can be linked to pelvic floor problems. For example, if we collapse our chest while sitting, we end up with a "C-curve" in the spine. I challenge you to try this while you are reading right now. This makes it difficult to take a deep breath, and as a consequence, the muscles of the pelvic floor don't receive the gentle "exercise" they need of stretching and contracting with every breath in and out.

In short, if your posture is not good and you're not taking in deep breaths to the abdomen, your pelvic floor is most definitely suffering. Everything is connected, and deep belly breathing is the most efficient way to take care of the pelvic floor.

It's not easy to change breathing habits and patterns, and the key is never to force. But to get you started on deepening the breath, here's a little exercise you can try.

Deepening the Breath:

1. Lie on your back with knees bent and feet hip-width apart.

2. To begin, take a few minutes to tune in to your body. Notice how you're feeling; notice areas with tension or tightness. Notice the movement of the breath, not judging or trying to change anything, just observing.

3. Put one hand on your lower belly below the navel, the other on your chest. Allow yourself to feel the breath move under your hands for a couple of minutes.

4. Then, as you exhale, gently contract the lower abdomen, moving the navel toward the spine. Repeat a few times, each time emptying out the air more fully. As you inhale, let the belly relax and soften. Allow the air to fill your lungs as the belly naturally inflates. Repeat three to five breaths; then just relax and return to your normal breath. Rest.

5. For round two, again draw the navel toward the spine as you exhale. As you get used to adding the sighing sound on the exhale, begin to add it on a small inhale as well; this will challenge the diaphragm and make the movement of the breath slightly deeper. Repeat this breath eight to ten times or as long as comfortable; then again, relax and return to your normal breath.

If you are someone who is noticing stiffness more frequently after exercise *and* stretching, then you will really benefit from a Pilates routine. Doing this simple breathing exercise a couple of times a day or at the start of the day will go a long way toward strengthening and engaging the diaphragm, and, in turn, it will slowly deepen your breath over time.

Find out more about Pilates specifically for women over 40 at www.level4pt.com/pilates.

CHAPTER 6

SCIATICA (LITERALLY, A PAIN IN THE BUTT!)

Mary's Story

I was going about my usual Sunday. I went to the gym to perform my regular exercise routine and then went to the grocery store immediately after. I was feeling great, and after unloading my groceries and putting away my laundry, all of a sudden, I felt a twinge on the right side of my lower back. I immediately knew something wasn't right.

I tried not to think too much about it and thought after a good night's sleep it would just go away on its own. But that wasn't the case.

I woke up in the morning unable to get out of bed without my husband's help. It was also extremely difficult to walk to the bathroom and even to put on my socks and shoes—not without struggling for 20 minutes anyway!.

It's been several weeks now, and I just can't seem to get rid of this annoying, burning, and excruciating pain that starts in my butt and runs down the back of my leg every time I take a step or bend forward. I now have difficulty sitting for more than ten minutes because the pain increases every time. Can you please help me?

Has a similar thing happened to you?

Unfortunately, I hear this story far too often from many of my clients. Just like Mary, many come to the wellness center in a great deal of pain wanting to know how to do the best sciatic pain treatment to get results at home.

Here's what happened when Mary came into our wellness center and was able to find out that a combination of incorrect lifting movements in the gym and incorrect lifting of heavy groceries and laundry basket at home, had caused something in her back to show that it had had enough. And like most people who come in to see me with low back pain, she brushed it off, hoping she'd wake up the next day as if it never had happened.

But the following day, her pain was *still there*.

It can sometimes be hard to see what you are doing wrong in your lifestyle because, well, it's your lifestyle.

Your daily routine is so well known to you that it can become second nature to lift things off the ground incorrectly, and that's what causes sciatic nerve pain.

Mary's back was still bad, but she decided to do nothing for it a little longer because she thought that by resting for a few more days, the pain would gradually go away.

But those days turned into weeks, and her back pain grew worse and worse—and the problem was that all of the sitting and resting she was doing to make it "better," was adding pressure to her back causing a shooting pain to run down her leg, which meant very little to no walking and even time off work.

Mary's condition is known as sciatica.

Sciatica pain symptoms are often so excruciating it makes it almost impossible to get out of the house, drive to shops, and even sleep comfortably. It nearly always gets worse when you sit.

Sciatica is a painful and life-limiting condition that requires seeking proper treatment sooner rather than later.

The sciatic nerve originates at the spinal cord, moves through the hips and buttocks, and divides and moves into both legs. It is one of the most critical *(and the longest)* nerves we have in the human body. It directly affects the sensations we feel in our legs and controls their movement.

The unmistakable symptoms of sciatica are very specific and usually appear in the form of pain that travels down through the lower back region, through the buttocks, and into the legs. Any movement that involves the lower back, hips, or legs tends to exacerbate the pain and cause more intense symptoms.

Many people also report a *"pins and needles"* sensation accompanied by uncomfortable tingling in the feet or toes. Others report weakness in the leg muscles and numbness in the feet and legs along the sciatic nerve route. Severe cases may result in a complete loss of movement and sensation in areas along the path that the sciatic nerve travels.

Although rare, in extreme cases, sciatica may also cause bladder or bowel incontinence. This complaint is symptomatic of Cauda Equina Syndrome (CES), where nerve roots in the spine can't send messages from the brain anymore due to swelling. This is one of the few instances where it is immediately necessary to consult with a medical doctor, but without changes in bowel/bladder function, weakness in the legs, or numbness or tingling in the saddle region between the legs, conservative treatment is the most EFFECTIVE method for long-lasting results.

What Causes Sciatica?

Several conditions related to the spinal cord and the nerves connected to it can cause sciatica. Some of the most common causes of sciatica we see at the clinic include:

Herniated discs: Cartilage separates the vertebrae of the spinal cord. These soft pads that protect the spine are composed of a thick material that allows flexibility and cushions movement. A herniated disc happens when the first cartilage layer is ruptured. The material within the disc then compresses the sciatic nerve and causes numbness and pain. Slipped discs are a common cause of sciatica in many of the patients we see.

Spondylolisthesis: This is another ailment associated with a degenerative *(worn)* disc. It occurs when a vertebra or spinal bone extends over another. This overlap then pinches the nerves leading to the sciatic nerve.

Spinal stenosis: also referred to as lumbar spinal stenosis, leads to narrowing of the lower part of the spinal canal. This narrowing exerts pressure on the spine as well as the sciatic nerve.

Piriformis syndrome: is one of the rarer neuromuscular ailments. The piriformis muscle *(that runs through your butt)* tightens or contracts involuntarily, leading to sciatica. The piriformis muscle links the lower spine to the thighbones. Sitting for long periods can exacerbate it. It's also susceptible to injury from falls, sports, or traffic collisions.

How We Diagnose Sciatica

First off, no two cases are the same. The symptoms of sciatica vary from one individual to another, depending on the cause of the inflammation. But I always start with your complete medical history to look for clues as to what caused your sciatic nerve to become injured or inflamed.

Next, I check for any adjacent injuries, areas of tenderness, or pain. Finally, I get you to describe the pain you feel, what makes it better and worse, and how it started initially.

The physical exam to check for sciatica includes testing the reflexes in your legs and measuring your muscle strength. I may also ask you to perform stretching and movement exercises to determine what type of movement increases your pain. As a physical therapist and musculoskeletal expert, my assessment to rule out a hip problem versus a back problem can help you reach a better diagnosis of where the pain may be originating.

Ninety-five percent of the time further testing with X-rays, MRIs, and nerve conduction tests are NOT necessary to ease sciatica symptoms. A physical therapist can provide many solutions to give you relief before considering an injection or surgery. Will your doctor tell you this? Not very often.

MOST cases of sciatica can be dealt with at your physical therapist's office—without the need to see a medical doctor.

How long should I wait before getting help?

If you or somebody you know has been struggling with any type of sciatica pain for more than ten days, it's very likely you'll run into the same problems Mary encountered. This will NOT go away magically on its own, although many people think it will! Suppose you want to avoid dangerous surgeries, medication with unpleasant side effects, and steroid injections. In that case, one of the best ways to treat sciatica is to undergo physical therapy with a therapist who specializes in treating sciatic nerve problems. A physical therapist can help you strengthen the back muscles and posture and help prevent future flare ups of sciatica.

In mild cases, you should be able to continue with your daily routine as much as possible. And this is key because inactivity and lying horizontally *(in front of Netflix)* can exacerbate the symptoms.

Here are some other helpful reminders if you are dealing with sciatica and what you can start doing immediately:

1. *Don't sit for longer than 20 minutes (as mentioned in Chapter 4).*

Sitting is the number one reason why sciatic pain is so common today because of the stress, strain, and pressure it creates on your back. The anatomy and structure of your back were not designed for prolonged sitting, which is often the "silent killer" that plagues most people with back and sciatica pain. If you find yourself having to work a desk job or spend a lot of time at home on the computer, try setting an alarm on your phone or computer, and stand up, just for 25 to 30 seconds every half hour. Moving periodically allows your body to reset itself and readjust. Your back needs a bit of pressure release every so often so that it does not get stuck in a singular position for too long.

2. *Don't try to exercise through pain.*

"No pain, no gain." Really? An often-overlooked downside of continuing to perform exercises that are painful is that it will automatically cause you to compensate by utilizing other muscles that aren't necessarily meant to take up that much load. This causes a downward spiral into habitual compensatory patterns and further injuries. By not performing the exercises in a pain-free range, you're basically not providing a healing environment for the injured sciatic nerve.

3. *Sleep with a pillow between your knees.*

As simple as it sounds (almost too simple), this is the tip that I give clients when they are having sciatic pain. Many report that sleeping with a pillow between their knees makes quite a difference.

By putting a pillow between your knees, it offsets the "pull" that your hip is placing on your back and sciatic nerve! This simple tip can reduce your pain by well over 20 percent within just one night!

4. *Stay hydrated.*

This is the BIG office worker mistake that could be zapping your energy. One really simple way to avoid this is to cut out the stuff that makes you dehydrated in the first place. Things like excessive coffee, tea, alcohol, and energy drinks will make you dehydrated as a consequence of drinking too much of them.

And being dehydrated can cause muscle aches, pains, and fatigue. So, it's important that you maintain a healthy water intake in order to eliminate any extra or unwanted tension in your muscles.

Our tip: drink sensible amounts of water often throughout the day.

For more helpful tips on sciatica, check out our sciatica guide online here: www.level4pt.com/sciatica.

CHAPTER 7

SEX HURTS! (DYSPAREUNIA)

Trisha was a 54-year-old who called seeking my advice. She had three C-sections about 15 years ago, then a laparoscopic surgery to remove her gallbladder a year ago. Her abdominals felt weak, she didn't have any complaints of back pain, and she had good bowel/bladder control. Her biggest complaint was about having pain when she attempted intercourse with her husband, but she thought that was just part of menopause.

She enjoyed sex before, but now it was creating a strain on their intimate relationship. She didn't know what to do.

After discussing this with her, I let her know an internal assessment would give me a better idea of why she was having so much discomfort. If she couldn't tolerate a pelvic exam, then we would work on strategies to be able to work up to it so she could ease the pain and tension in her pelvic muscles.

With a pelvic floor assessment, I was able to check if she had any tender trigger point areas; her muscles appeared strong and able to relax when I gave her some cuing.

Then I had her do a couple of breathing exercises to see if I could teach her how to relax her pelvic floor muscles a little more. It was a quick assessment, followed by instructions for what she needed to do to make a difference in relaxing her pelvic muscles over the next few weeks with specific yoga-based relaxation and stretching exercises and a few physical therapy sessions for some hands-on release of the pelvic floor muscles.

She was happy to have a full description of WHY she was uncomfortable during sex, and she now had a PLAN to know what she needed to do to improve. Trisha saw me for six visits total; together, we not only cured her painful sex issue, but we fixed some chronic hip pain she had felt over the last ten years!

This is just one example to give you an idea of the power of having the right guidance.

Unfortunately, as you may be all too aware, causes of painful sex are commonly misdiagnosed or not diagnosed at all by primary care providers. Often, women just endure the pain and uncomfortable feeling they experience during a gynecological exam, or the doctor encourages them to "just relax." An internal exam or sexual intercourse should *not* be painful (and you shouldn't have to use medication like a vaginal diazepam to mask the pain).

If pain is experienced, then it is highly related to the pelvic floor muscle's function, which is creating increased tension in that area. This IS a muscular problem that needs intervention, so you really don't have to struggle with it for the rest of your life and cause a strain on your relationship.

Some women have pain during sex for months or even years after childbirth. And some have chronic pain, itching, or burning in their vulva—the tissue surrounding the opening of the vagina.

What exactly caused Trisha's pain? A restricted, painful pelvic floor has a variety of causes. Sometimes, the type of activity you are accustomed to over many years can lead to it. Commonly, ballet dancers, gymnasts, ice skaters, and equestrians are more often the ones with this issue earlier in life. This can be attributed to their inherent need to focus on posture and muscle control to perform their sport, sometimes overtraining so much that the internal muscles haven't learned how to release and could be firing "ON" 24/7.

Another cause can be emotional or physical trauma/abuse, which has now created a subconscious holding of the pelvic floor muscles, creating pain like it would with any other muscle that is constantly contracting. Abdominal or pelvic surgery can also cause issues. Think about a tight muscle in your back; you get tension and pain and feel like you want to stretch it out for relief.

Many times, women are subconsciously tense in their pelvic floor, and they are unable to recognize how to relax it. They need to be given verbal and tactile cues to have the awareness to ease it.

Additionally, during midlife, vaginal dryness can be the leading cause of painful intercourse. Before menopause, the walls of the vagina typically have a thin layer of moisture on them. This moisture is secreted by the cells of the vaginal walls and helps sperm survive and travel. It also reduces friction during sexual intercourse.

When estrogen production starts to decline in menopause, vaginal secretions and moisture lessen, and vaginal dryness may occur.

Symptoms of vaginal dryness may include:

- irritation, burning, or itching
- lowered sex drive
- post-sex bleeding
- recurring urinary tract infections

Vaginal dryness can cause discomfort and painful intercourse, and it can negatively affect quality of life.

There are things you can do to help reduce pain during sex and add lubrication to the vaginal area:

- **Vaginal moisturizers or lubricants** add moisture to and around the vagina. They can be inserted for internal moisture or applied to the vulva.

- **A vaginal dilator** can help stretch and enlarge the vagina if tightening occurs. This should be tried under the guidance of a physical therapist to ensure proper use.

- **Pelvic floor exercises** can also help strengthen and relax certain vaginal muscles, which can also bring more blood flow and circulation to the area to increase the amount of natural lubrication (very effective and natural!).

With the proper guidance of a pelvic floor physical therapist, the goal is to gently stretch this area and release trigger points that are causing pain. This can be uncomfortable, particularly if you have chronic pain or aren't keen on the idea of internal massage. But a practitioner with whom you feel comfortable will guide you the right way so you don't have to suffer with the problem any longer.

(Try the exercises to lengthen and stretch the pelvic floor in the BONUS section!)

I have recently had clients who have undergone a C-section or hysterectomy and are experiencing this type of tension, which could be due to the restriction in the lower abdominal region, area sensitivity, and guarding because of the scar. Being instructed on stretching and relaxing techniques that are safe and effective after six weeks post-op can make a world of difference for this specific issue.

You should have a sense of release or relief afterward when the tightness eases. For a lot of my clients, it may just take a few treatments to work through this internally with some manual therapy and soft tissue mobilization techniques. I then follow it up with specific relaxation exercises, yoga poses, and breath work that address the pelvic floor and allow it to gain long-term relief naturally.

No woman should have to deal with pain during intimacy or during a gynecological exam.

If your muscles are in a subconscious state of contracting and they haven't been taught how to relax, then it is not possible for it to just happen on its own without professional guidance!

If you have specific concerns or want to find out more, please visit www.level4pt.com/pelvic-pain (free guide download), or listen to Episode 15 on the *Women's Health Happy Hour Podcast* (available wherever you listen to podcasts).

CHAPTER 8

PELVIC ORGAN PROLAPSE— BREAKING THE SILENCE

Veronica is a 61-year-old female who had been feeling increased pressure and heaviness in her pelvic area. She wanted to stay active but was concerned symptoms would worsen and would continue to affect her as she reached her late 60s and 70s. She was even experiencing cramp-like feelings in her lower abdominal region, and it made her anxious because she didn't know the cause.

After multiple visits, her doctor told her that she had a prolapse and gave her the option of using a device called a pessary that would help hold it in place. The pessary was very uncomfortable, and she decided to do some research on her own, which led her to read about pelvic floor physical therapy. Veronica had been working on Kegel exercises with little change in her symptoms over the past year. Her kids were now in their 20s, and she asked me, "Isn't it too late for me? I was told surgery could fix this."

An assessment revealed she had a very weak pelvic floor and was unable to activate her muscles without compensating with her glutes and inner thighs. Additionally, every Kegel contraction she performed caused her to push out her abdominals and hold her breath.

We worked on correcting this for the next few weeks, and I gave her cuing and targeted exercises to work on between sessions. In a short amount of time, she was so relieved to have a renewed sense of confidence about her body. The cramping symptoms went away, her back felt even stronger, and she experienced no more heaviness/pressure in the pelvic area. She said it really was amazing, and she was sorry she had waited so long to come get my help!

Why is Veronica's story so common? I hear this time and time again—women who go about life thinking this is just the way it has to be, not taking action to help themselves. The reason I included Veronica's story was to show you that it can happen to women of all ages, and conservative interventions can make a world of difference.

Some women consider living with pelvic organ prolapse to feel like they are carrying a little ball around in their underwear or like a tampon is slipping out. It sounds dramatic—if you haven't experienced it. Still, this description perfectly illustrates the unrelenting pressure and tugging pain inside the vagina that accompanies this common women's health complaint. But, actually, women tell us it's the psychological weight of the condition that weighs heaviest.

> Many women report a fear of sex, have low back or lower abdominal pain, and the need to pee ALL the time.
> *It's miserable.*

But perhaps the worst feeling of all when you're dealing with a pelvic organ prolapse is the sensation that your insides are going to fall out, which makes you not want to walk, work, exercise, or socialize.

If you are one of the unlucky ones with severe symptoms, it may surprise you to learn that some women don't experience any symptoms and only learn they have a prolapse when they see their doctor for an annual Pap smear. Or, worse still, their first clue about having a prolapse is when they see or feel a lump or bulge in or protruding from their vagina or anus.

But even without symptoms, "prolapse" is not the news any woman wants to hear. It can be pretty horrifying if you haven't experienced it before.

But it doesn't have to be scary. It's not a life sentence either. It's very treatable—with the proper support. *You can get your life back.*

The term *pelvic organ prolapse* refers to one or more of your pelvic organs, such as the uterus, bowel, or bladder, sliding down and bulging into or outside of your vaginal canal or anus. But it's a bit of a catch-all name because this condition can present itself in so many different ways. It's not one thing, and every woman is different.

For instance, the most common version of pelvic organ prolapse is when the bladder prolapses into the vagina. We call this a cystocele. But this is most definitely not the only type of prolapse. You may also suffer from vaginal vault prolapse, uterine prolapse, urethrocele, enterocele, or rectocele.

Vaginal vault prolapse occurs when the upper section of the vagina falls into the vaginal canal or protrudes out of the vagina. It is common after full or partial hysterectomy.

Uterine prolapse happens when the womb moves down from its usual position and encroaches into the vaginal canal. In severe cases, uterine tissue may protrude outside the vagina. This type of prolapse is most commonly due to the pressure of pregnancy, excess weight, or repetitive coughing.

Urethrocele is where the urethra, the tube that transports urine out of the body, protrudes into the vaginal canal. This condition is most commonly associated with childbirth as the baby moves through the birth canal. It usually occurs in tandem with a cystocele, a bladder prolapse, but it can happen independently.

Enterocele occurs when the small bowel descends into the lower pelvis area and puts pressure on the top of the vagina, creating a lump inside or outside of the vagina. Like all prolapses, an enterocele forms when the pelvic floor muscles lose strength, but it can be brought on by constipation, straining, and coughing.

Rectocele is where the rectum bulges forward into the vaginal wall.

Without professional consultation, it's hard to know which of these specific types of prolapse you're suffering from. They all cause similar symptoms like pelvic pain and pressure and problems urinating or trouble with your bowels. Effective treatment for all types of pelvic organ prolapse starts with proper diagnosis because treatment protocols differ for each one.

Sadly, pelvic organ prolapse sometimes slips under the radar. It can go undiagnosed and untreated because it's often confused with other conditions like urinary stress incontinence and overactive bladder. The prolapse causes similar symptoms like increased urination, leakage, and a failure to empty the bladder properly.

Seeing a doctor first may be helpful to rule out any other red flags or health conditions, but just know it is not always necessary. Very often, women discover their prolapse and start "googling" their symptoms, then come see someone like me first to confirm it if they haven't seen their doctor. We can then get straight to work on improving the symptoms, especially if surgery does not sound like something you want to jump into (or even need!). Also, there are so many women that end up finding someone like me after their doctor told them surgery would be the only option. I just want to let women know that there is a high probability that you may not actually need surgery if you work on the root cause with a pelvic floor physical therapist. I have even saved women from needing surgery in the long run!

What Causes Pelvic Organ Prolapse?

Pelvic organ prolapse is most likely to occur when the pelvic floor muscles have become weakened. They're no longer able to hold the pelvic organs in place effectively.

Some genetic conditions and inherited connective tissue disorders can cause this muscle weakness, such as Benign Hypermobility Syndrome, Ehlers-Danos Syndrome (EDS), or Marfan Syndrome. But these conditions are rare.

In most cases, pelvic floor weakness results from wear and tear, hysterectomy, or vaginal childbirth, particularly in long labors, difficult births, and with large babies. It may also stem from excess weight, repetitive strain, heavy lifting, bowel resection, gynecological cancers, other abdominal surgeries, or even chronic constipation. In other words, anything that puts prolonged pressure on the abdomen and pelvic organs can cause pelvic floor weakness.

How to Ease Symptoms of Pelvic Organ Prolapse

Well, the first thing to understand is that a pelvic organ prolapse tends to worsen over time. It won't go away or fix itself, so I recommend you not delay getting treatment to give yourself the best chance of full resolution.

Depending on the severity of the prolapse and its effect on your daily life, your doctor may recommend corrective surgery. The various surgical options to lift and repair major pelvic organ prolapses include vaginal mesh surgery, a complete hysterectomy, or, in the most severe cases, closing the vagina.

All of these options should be a last resort. They require lots of downtime. You'll need up to 12 weeks off work, and you'll need to refrain from sex and using tampons and other sanitary protection in that time, too. As with all surgeries, these also carry a risk of serious complications, but your doctor will help you decide whether the surgical route is right for you. The benefits may outweigh the risks if the prolapse is severe enough to warrant it.

But suppose your pelvic organ prolapse is a mild to moderate case? In that case, non-surgical treatment may be the best and least invasive option. This treatment includes lifestyle changes, losing weight, and treating chronic constipation with a high fiber diet, if necessary.

You could also consider using latex vaginal pessaries inserted into the vagina to bolster your pelvic floor muscles and provide extra support for your pelvic organs and prevent damage to the vaginal wall.

The most common type of vaginal pessary for pelvic organ prolapse is called a ring pessary, which you can insert and remove yourself. You can also still have sex while wearing a ring pessary, although lots of women prefer to remove and reinsert. This non-surgical device, and others like it, are a good option when you need additional support but would like to have more children. In this case, you want to avoid radical surgery or hysterectomy.

Vaginal pessaries are safe and non-invasive, but they're not without risks from infection, allergic reactions, or irritation. If you've ever had an allergy to latex, they may not be suitable for you.

After menopause, some women find that supplementary estrogen, as a pill, patch, pessary, or cream, can ease some of the factors like vaginal dryness and the associated painful intercourse that can make pelvic organ prolapse worse. But hormone replacement therapy is not for everyone. As with surgery, you need to weigh the pros and cons.

Physical therapy and specific pelvic floor exercises have proven to be highly beneficial for mild to moderate pelvic organ prolapses.

Check out more tips about pelvic organ prolapse here: www.level4pt.com/pelvic-organ-prolapse.

CHAPTER 9

HEALING AFTER HYSTERECTOMY

Have you had a hysterectomy, or are you scheduled to have one?

Are you wondering what to expect and how to heal well afterward?

A hysterectomy is the second most common medical procedure for women in the US after the C-Section. Studies reveal that more than 600,000 women undergo this procedure annually across the US. It involves the removal of the cervix and the uterus via surgery.[4]

Most women that opt for hysterectomies are women of the age group of 60 and above. However, many younger women also undergo this procedure because of conditions like endometriosis or because of cancerous or precancerous cells in or around the womb, or when there is a medical risk of developing cancer in the womb.

After a hysterectomy, doctors recommend not undertaking anything strenuous (such as lifting weights above ten pounds) and abstaining from physical intimacy for a minimum of six weeks. These guidelines give the tissues time to heal while ensuring you don't strain your pelvic floor muscles and rupture the stitches.

4

A hysterectomy is a big deal—from a physical and a psychological perspective. Significant hormone changes send you off on an emotional rollercoaster and cause a whole host of uncomfortable symptoms, such as vaginal dryness and painful sex, incontinence, and pelvic pain. It's major abdominal surgery.

You need adequate (almost total) rest directly after the surgery, too, followed by a gradual increase in activity after the period of recuperation recommended by your surgeon.

But don't worry—you can take several steps to prevent or minimize the physical symptoms and make sure you have the proper emotional support.

The word *hysterectomy* describes the medical removal of the uterus or "womb." In some cases, the operation removes the uterus in isolation, but in other cases, the surgeon may suggest removing additional parts of the female reproductive system at the same time.

The exact procedure depends on your specific situation and medical symptoms, as dictated by healthcare professionals.

But you are likely to undergo one of these types of hysterectomy:

Subtotal hysterectomy: In this procedure, only the uterus is removed. Your cervix remains in its original place.

Laparoscopic hysterectomy: During this procedure, the surgeon makes tiny cuts or incisions to insert a miniature camera into your abdomen to view the inside of your pelvic region. The surgeon then removes your uterus via the vagina. This type of hysterectomy is minimally invasive, thanks to keyhole surgery. Also, recovery is usually quicker than an abdominal hysterectomy.

Radical or Wertheim's hysterectomy: This radical procedure involves removing a part of the vagina, the cervix, fallopian tubes, and uterus. This type of hysterectomy is usually only performed in the event of cancerous cells being present in order to prevent the disease from spreading to other parts of the body.

Vaginal hysterectomy: If you have a vaginal hysterectomy, your surgeon will remove your cervix and uterus via the vagina.

Total abdominal hysterectomy: Although this procedure is described as "total," unlike a radical hysterectomy where all the female reproductive system organs are removed, a total hysterectomy is limited to the removal of the uterus and the cervix.

One of the best resources for pre-op and post-op care for a hysterectomy— a pelvic floor physical therapist—is not usually recommended by the surgeon, but that is why I wrote this book, right? If what I have written can help just ten more women, it would be a success because I have witnessed firsthand the worry, frustration, and lack of guidance women are given when it comes to preparing for and recovering from a hysterectomy.

Pelvic floor physical therapy is beneficial pre- and post-hysterectomy to prevent and treat side effects that may occur because of the surgery, such as lower abdominal pressure, pain, incontinence, or prolapse.

For this type of therapy, many doctors won't even recommend seeing a physical therapist after the surgery, but this is an untapped resource that can help you heal with more confidence as well as promote a successful surgery! And in the case of pre-hysterectomy physical therapy, it potentially allows you to prevent any complaints from happening at all.

After undergoing a hysterectomy, the pelvic region generally is inflamed and irritated. This inflammation directly impacts the all-important pelvic floor muscles. They cannot contract or relax properly. They can also become taut as a protective mechanism to protect the inflamed tissues.

Even after the healing process has been completed and the tissues return to their pre-inflammatory state, it's not unusual for the pelvic floor muscles to remain dysfunctional, leading to chronic issues with urinary stress incontinence or consistent pain in the pelvic region.

If you haven't had your hysterectomy, yet, you can prevent these complications from arising and recover quicker with early intervention physical therapy. Either in preparation for your surgery or as soon as possible after your immediate rest period, a pelvic floor physical therapist can diagnose issues with your pelvic floor muscles and work with you to correct them before they start causing problems.

But even if it has been decades since you had your hysterectomy, you can still resolve these issues with physical therapy.

Physical Therapy Before Hysterectomy

Before surgery, I recommend a combination of the following:

- Specialized pelvic floor physical therapy and exercises to support the pelvic floor
- Resistance exercises to strengthen the upper and lower body
- Cardiovascular activities like cycling and walking
- Hydrotherapy
- Exercises for the transverse abdominals (those deep abdominal muscles that crunches won't help!)

After your hysterectomy surgery and the immediate rest period, you may experience the following symptoms:

- Inflammation and swelling in the pelvic region
- Diminished cardiovascular fitness and strength
- Pelvic pain

- Desensitization of the surgical area due to nerve involvement (temporary)
- Bruising
- Scar tissue

Everyone is different, however, so you may have completely different symptoms than the ones listed above. Still, these are the most common complaints women report after undergoing hysterectomy surgery.

Physical Therapy After Hysterectomy

After your surgery, you may remain in the hospital for four to seven days, subject to the type of procedure you opt for and the recommended recovery period. Once discharged, however, it is beneficial to begin pelvic floor physical therapy at the earliest possible point, as advised by your doctor.

Recovery Week One

Every woman is different—and your specific set of symptoms after surgery is likely to be different from someone else's. But the following might be part of your physical therapy treatment in the first week after your immediate recovery period:

- Gentle breathing exercises and engagement of the deep abdominals by small contractions performed in sync with breathing
- Pain control treatment
- Light range of movement exercises to move the legs and encourage blood flow and circulation
- Recommendations about the most appropriate sitting and standing positions to minimize pain and symptoms
- Advice on scar management
- Basic mobility exercises to prevent muscle stiffness

Recovery Weeks Two to Six

By this point, there should be a noticeable decrease in your symptoms. You should also notice that you can slowly return to your daily routine—with some thoughtful modifications.

During this time, your physical therapy treatment schedule might look something like this:

- Increasing the strengthening exercises
- An increase in transverse abdominal exercises
- Steadily increasing pelvic floor exercises in different positions
- Expanding the range of movement to strengthen the upper body
- Adding functional activities over time

Approximately six weeks after your hysterectomy, with effective guidance from a pelvic floor physical therapist, you should be able to resume all regular activities with no or minimal pain.

By the seventh week, it should be easier to carry moderate weights without any pain. Keep in mind that every woman is different, and what feels fine for one person may not be appropriate for you. Listening to your body and not pushing through any pain or discomfort should be your guide.

We don't just tell you to do 100 Kegels!

Post-hysterectomy self-care

Over the last decade, I've been able to narrow down what really does and doesn't work when it comes to easing issues that occur after hysterectomy.

1. *Six weeks may not be enough time to feel "normal" again.*

Oftentimes after surgery, including hysterectomies, surgeons provide a six-week timeline for recovery and a safe return to previous activities.

Unfortunately, this one-size-fits-all approach is not appropriate for all cases; what seems like normal activity or job duties for you, may be entirely different for another person.

Even though a hysterectomy is viewed as a routine surgery, it is still physical trauma for your body that requires time to heal. It is important to discuss with your surgeon at post-operative visits what full recovery means to you, and then plan accordingly for additional time off from work, sex, or exercise so that you can heal completely.

2. You might have urinary leakage or changes in urinary frequency.

After recovering from a hysterectomy, many women are horrified and embarrassed to find that they are now experiencing urinary incontinence with activities that never bothered them before, such as coughing, exercise, or laughing.

When the uterus and other organs are removed from the body, the pressure and support that was placed on the bladder and urethra changes. With more free space in the abdominal cavity, changes in force that occur during certain body movements now push directly on the bladder, causing you to be more likely to leak urine with activity.

The good news is that despite having a hysterectomy, you do not have to be doomed with leakage. As you learned in Chapter 3, the pelvic floor muscles that support the bladder and urethra can be trained to assist with and prevent leakage.

3. Sex might feel different (or be painful).

Despite the necessity of having a hysterectomy due to various reasons, the body still finds the surgical removal of an organ (or organs) to be very traumatizing. For this reason, many times after surgery, when a woman has healed and is able to resume her sex life, she notices that there are changes in the sensations she experiences during intercourse.

Sometimes, women simply are experiencing dryness due to changes in hormone levels that happen after removal of the uterus. Unfortunately, many women also note feeling pain that they previously did not experience with their partner. This is usually caused by overactivity of the pelvic floor muscles that become tight and restricted in an effort to protect the pelvic area after surgery.

However, this can be problematic as this tightness in the pelvic floor does not go away on its own and can affect your sex life and relationship. Internal assessment and treatment with a pelvic floor physical therapist, deep breathing exercises, and hip stretches can help relax those muscles and reteach your body how to enjoy sex again.

4. *You could develop a prolapsed bladder.*

A prolapse is a condition where the uterus, rectum, or bladder push on the vaginal wall, causing a feeling of fullness or heaviness in the vagina. Sometimes this bulge can be seen or felt by the woman or her partner.

After a surgery that results in removal of the uterus, there is less natural support for the colon, cervix, and bladder. As a result, these tissues "fall" downward, causing increased pressure within the vagina.

While prolapse can be very scary after a hysterectomy, it is important to note that it can be prevented with expert guidance to teach you how to use your core and pelvic floor muscles to help lift, exercise, and move correctly without the risk of damage and prolapse of the pelvic organs. This is not something to scare you or cause alarm, but the lack of support from your pelvic floor muscles can cause extra pressure or discomfort in the vaginal area, and this is a precursor to actually developing a prolapse.

So, those are some of the issues or changes your surgeon may not tell you about that could arise during recovery from a hysterectomy. Truth is, without knowing about your full history or type of hysterectomy or surgery that you had, I cannot tell you which of these may or may not happen to you. The key is that being prepared and understanding your own body can be the biggest factors in returning to 100 percent. A helpful free webinar that I offer periodically throughout the year on post-hysterectomy recovery can be found here: www.level4pt.com/events.

As a bonus, here are two effective post-surgical exercises that promote healing.

Post-surgical breathing:

Soon after surgery, you will most likely be instructed to take deep breaths several times per day to prevent pneumonia or other post-surgical complications. To practice this (unless your doctor specified otherwise), lie on your back, or wherever you are most comfortable, and place a hand on your abdomen and chest. Inhale through your nose, focusing on gently expanding your ribs and abdomen. Exhale out your mouth, and everything "comes in." Perform this ten times morning, noon, and night focusing on staying relaxed and pain free.

Rolling in bed:

Even with minimally invasive surgeries that have few stitches or little "downtime," moving your body after surgery can be painful. Moving and getting comfortable in bed can be one of the most difficult things! To combat this, when you want to roll in bed, perform a log roll. Start by lying on your back, and, one at a time, bend both knees to place your feet closer to your buttocks (you may also want to put a pillow between your knees, or hold a pillow to your abdomen if you have stitches). As you exhale, roll your head, shoulders, hips, and knees to their desired side as a unit at the same time. To sit up in bed, simply press down with your top hand on the bed to lift your torso as your legs come off of the bed at the same time.

CHAPTER 10

THE DREADED WEIGHT GAIN

As hormones shift over 40 and beyond, weight gain is a very common complaint among women. Contributing factors can include stress, lack of exercise and activity, a shift in our hormone levels, and chronic inflammation.

Dealing with chronic inflammation can lead to disease, weight gain, and more harmful effects on our body. Nutrition and exercise can't go without mentioning in this book because women's bodies need more attention as they grow older.

As women age, they become more fragile and more susceptible to injury and chronic illness. For example, blood vessels tend to get stiffer, causing the heart to work harder to pump blood at an appropriate rate. Bones tend to shrink in size and density, making them weaker and more susceptible to fracture. And muscles generally lose some of their strength, endurance, and flexibility.

But changes that come with age are possible to slow down, and nothing we do to improve our health is ever too little— and it is never too late, no matter when we start! We can make choices that improve our ability to maintain an active life, do the things we enjoy, and spend time with those we love.

What your doctor might not tell you is that changing (improving) your lifestyle with diet and exercise actually improves your brain, too!

Once you know why you want to make healthy changes in your life, the next step is to decide how you're going to achieve those changes!

It's easy for life to get in the way sometimes, so you have to figure out what works for you. Weight gain after menopause can feel inevitable, but if you are mindful about what you eat, it doesn't have to be.

Whether you're just starting to go through perimenopause or have already bid a fond farewell to your last period, it is never too late to get your eating back on track. Because I have been going through this journey myself, I find these tips to be very helpful—and this is the advice you WON'T get from your medical doctor who might not have studied nutrition and exercise in medical school. You can't expect to go through hormonal changes and NOT address your nutrition and activity as a way to improve your aches/pains, change your body composition, and fight chronic diseases such as diabetes and hypertension!

How Changes in Hormones Affect Metabolism

During perimenopause, progesterone levels decline slowly and steadily, while estrogen levels fluctuate greatly from day to day and even within the same day. Later in perimenopause, when menstrual cycles become more irregular, the ovaries produce very little estrogen. They produce even less during menopause.

From puberty until perimenopause, women tend to store fat in their hips and thighs as subcutaneous fat. Although it can be hard to lose, this type of fat doesn't increase disease risk very much. However, during menopause, low estrogen levels promote fat storage in the belly area as visceral fat, which is linked to insulin resistance, type 2 diabetes, heart disease, and other health problems. Hormone level changes may only be one contributing factor to weight gain during menopause. More frequently, older women gain weight due to less activity and have less muscle mass, which means they burn fewer calories during the day. These factors can all increase a woman's risk for weight gain and increased body fat during the transition to menopause.

Six Tips for Peri- and Postmenopausal Weight Loss

1. *Look at the big picture!* You can't stop your metabolism from slowing down, but that is rarely the only factor contributing to weight gain. Maybe knee pain is interfering with your exercise plans, or maybe your busy caregiving schedule doesn't leave much energy for planning and cooking healthy meals. By identifying the hurdles to a healthier lifestyle, you can brainstorm ways to clear them.

2. *Keep track.* It's easy to lose track of the chips you munch mindlessly in front of the TV or not realize how much oatmeal you're eating every morning. A food journal can help you keep tabs on how much you're really eating and identify reasonable places to cut back.

3. *Focus on healthy calories.* Build your meals around healthy calories like lean proteins and veggies. Try to cut back on the not-so-healthy fare. It can be harder to burn starchy carbs like bread, pasta, and baked goods, so be mindful of cutting back or avoiding those. Beverages, too, are often a source of sneaky calories. To cut back, reach for sparkling water in place of wine or soda. Add a splash of milk to brewed coffee instead of ordering a latte.

4. *Structure your meals.* Eating regular meals and healthy snacks will help you keep weight off and feel more satisfied. Don't skip meals or try fad diets. Those can further slow down your metabolism and make it even harder to lose weight. Try to have your bigger meals earlier in the day, so you'll have more time to burn calories before you hit the pillow.

5. *Try intermittent fasting* (my personal favorite as I have found this fairly easy to do). While skipping meals outright is a no-go, some people have success with intermittent fasting (listen to Episode 34 of my podcast *Women's Health Happy Hour*). Try to eat all your healthy goal calories within an 8-hour window (for example, from 10 a.m. to 6 p.m.). Outside those hours, stick to water, tea, and black coffee. This type of eating pattern can help you burn calories more efficiently and has shown effects of decreasing inflammation and the insulin response.

6. *Ask for help.* If you've made healthy lifestyle changes and the scale isn't budging, talk to your doctor. There may be other reasons for weight gain, such as thyroid problems, medication side effects, or depression, so you'll want to rule out other causes.

A registered dietitian can also help figure out a sustainable way of eating to avoid putting on unwanted pounds as you age.

We all strive to be healthier, and it's easy to get discouraged when starting a new fitness regimen or trying to lose weight. Why? Well, because you can hit weight loss plateaus and feel frustrated when the number on the scale doesn't go down as fast as you had hoped. But getting in shape isn't just about a number—it's about your overall health. It means having more energy AND being able to fit into your favorite jeans.

Instead of constantly obsessing over those three numbers, you will be PROUD of the positive changes within your body that come from making healthier choices. You will strive to get a better understanding of how to avoid the same mistakes over and over each year.

Don't let your scale dictate your mood when your great health is so much more than just a number.

Here are five ways you can track your progress after throwing your bathroom scales out the window:

1. Energy Levels

Taking note of whether you feel sluggish can be a good indicator of your overall health. Chances are, if you're eating healthy, drinking plenty of water, and exercising daily, you'll be feeling the benefits. You'll feel more alert, have a better night's sleep, and won't suffer from that afternoon slump so many women feel.

Feeling healthy is the first step in looking and feeling your best. So, don't brush off the inside-out effects of your new lifestyle, even if weight loss is your main goal.

2. Sleep

Humans spend close to a third of their lives sleeping, and when they get enough rest…they feel great! It's a fact that people need sleep for physical, mental, and emotional health. The number of hours you sleep is important, but the *quality* of sleep is VITAL. If you're unable to get a good night's sleep, it could be a sign that you're not experiencing great health and fitness. You have probably heard for years now that frequent aerobic exercise can lead to a better night's sleep, warding off insomnia and boosting your energy levels during the day.

Also, cutting down on alcohol and stimulants like caffeine before bed should help you drift off easier. Or, consider making time for yourself with a quick yoga routine before you switch the lights off.

If you are getting quality sleep, that's a great sign that you're doing something right. Remember, how you start the day is just as important as how you end it.

3. Mood

Did you know that your mood is closely linked to healthy eating (aka fueling your body)? Of course, everyone has days when they feel worn out from a busy week at work or when the kids are home during a break from school. In general, healthy people are able to bounce back, feel good, and maintain a fair amount of energy.

If you're in a good mood, that's great! It can be a reflection of good health. But, on the other hand, if you're feeling a little low, or you've got a short fuse, this can be a sign that it's time to make some lifestyle changes. Losing your temper can happen when blood sugar is low, so eating balanced meals is key. Also, adding more exercise into your week can help release those feel-good chemicals.

4. Strength

As women age, the number on the scale seems LESS relevant than the ability to DO MORE. Strength equals the ability to maintain your self-worth, independence, and stamina! When you start a new exercise regimen that includes weight training, you *want* to add muscle. That's right! As mentioned previously, the more muscle mass you have, the more calories you will burn. This affects your ability to improve your metabolism and look more toned.

And while that muscle might register on the scale as increased weight and lead you to think you're not seeing results, you can actually lose fat *and* gain muscle at the same time—it's the ideal scenario! You'll notice your jeans fitting better, and you will have more energy and BE STRONGER.

When you're able to do more activities throughout the day or lift more weight in your workout sessions as the weeks go by, your body is getting stronger. Let your newfound strength empower you! You can now do MORE with your body than you once could, and that's amazing!

5. Skin Complexion

You may have spent money on creams and lotions to keep your skin looking younger, when younger-looking skin is often a natural byproduct of exercise. How your skin looks can also reflect what's going on inside your body. Did you know that your skin is the biggest organ in the body? When you don't get enough exercise, it can start to show on your face—literally.

Here's a little-known secret: people over 40 who exercise frequently have skin closer in composition to that of 20- and 30-year-olds. That's right! When you start to take care of your inner health, it often affects your outer beauty as well. Even having more energy and simply feeling better can make us glow from the inside out—and that's something to smile about.

But regardless of age, skin problems can be signs that indicate you're not experiencing great health. Two of the most common signs are paleness and itchy skin.

So, pay attention to how radiant (or not so radiant) your skin looks, and switch up your lifestyle habits if need be. The scale shows weight, but it doesn't measure how much better you look and feel, if you can walk the stairs without losing your breath, how strong you're becoming, or if you can play with your kids or grandkids for hours.

On your fitness journey, don't let the number on the scale rule your life and how you feel. If the number on the scale isn't moving, consider first how your new, healthier choices are making you feel. Do you have more energy? A more positive mood? How are your clothes fitting? Are you getting stronger and being able to do more without feeling like you are out of breath? Judge your progress by "health," instead. You'll learn how to listen to your body, and your efforts will pay off.

Fill out an inquiry form at www.level4pt.com to request more information about our virtual women's health nutrition counseling programs!

CHAPTER 11

BEST WAYS TO STAY FIT DURING PERI- & POSTMENOPAUSE

Congratulations! If you've been following my advice thus far, you are already way ahead of the majority of women in our society today who are suffering with chronic aches and pains, having unnecessary surgeries, and relying on medications instead of living a healthy, happy, and active lifestyle like they deserve.

How can I be so sure you'll get a positive result? Well, because the most effective way to live a healthy, happy, and active lifestyle and fight the "symptoms" that are typically associated with a stereotypical downward spiral of aging as a female are the methods outlined in this book. When you are doing the right things for your health, you feel more energetic and youthful.

Now, that's not to say you can't do even better. You can definitely say "it's never too late" by paying a bit more attention to some overlooked daily activities that could make you look and feel better than you have in at least five years—and people will notice.

This chapter will show you the best and most proven methods that can benefit your physical health as a female in your middle age and beyond. I will explain in more depth the importance of increasing flexibility, why

Pilates is my top recommendation for low-impact exercise, the benefits of the often overlooked exercise of walking, and the necessity for strength training. These easy, practical, and natural ways to stay active will make you move easier, bend further, stretch more…and ache much less.

When Was the Last Time You Could Touch Your Toes?

Without some degree of flexibility, life will be a bit more difficult than you might like, and if you're 40 or over, you're probably already beginning to lose flexibility on a daily basis. As you begin to lose flexibility in muscles and joints (Have you tried touching your toes lately?), you'll notice increasing difficulty with the simplest of things, such as putting on your socks and shoes, getting in and out of the car without a struggle, and even doing some simple household chores.

Those next day aches and pains, the ones you feel after an active day spent walking or doing things in the garden, are caused by lack of flexibility, too. So, if you recognize an increasing lack of flexibility in yourself, it might help to know a little bit about why it's happening and what you can do about it.

The problem is that not many people are open to the idea that you can increase flexibility, as if stiffness and a lack of freedom of choice when it comes to movement are an inevitable age thing. And, sure, they are—to some degree! But that doesn't mean you can't slow down these effects or even reverse them.

I hear it all the time from clients who first come into the wellness center saying they've never been flexible their entire lives, but then I find out that they've never worked at building flexibility. It's comparable to brushing your teeth once, and then expecting to have great oral hygiene for the rest of your life. Having great flexibility is no different; like brushing your teeth, you have to make it a daily habit. So, here is the big question: How do you reduce the impact of muscles and joints that get stiffer and tighter by the day?

It's really simple: don't stop moving!

The temptation is to think that because you're feeling tighter and stiffer, you should stop and wait for the stiffness to go away on its own. More often than not, that's the worst thing you can do, and rarely does it do anything other than get worse.

Implementing low-impact exercises like walking, cycling, and swimming is a great way to prevent flexibility problems in your later years—even if you only do them for 30 to 40 minutes, three times a week. An added benefit of being active is that it facilitates stretching.

When you finish exercising, before you plop on the couch, stretch the muscles you usually feel tightness in the most. At this point, immediately after a nice exercise session, your body is in the best state it can possibly be to stretch out your muscles because it is warm. It's so much easier and safer to stretch muscles and joints when you're warm.

Why Flexibility Can Slow Down Aging

Are you finding it difficult to sit on low couches, chairs, the toilet, or on the floor? Are you waking up every morning with a stiff back? Are your shoulders beginning to round forward? Is putting on your socks and shoes becoming more difficult? Can you not touch your toes from a standing position?

If you're saying to yourself, "That's not me because I'm more of an active type of individual," then I'm not letting you get away that easy.

Let's really think about this: Are you finding it more difficult to reach down to pick up your kids or grandkids? Is it becoming more difficult to get in and out of your car? Are you wondering why other people in the gym are making exercises look so easy and aren't plagued with injuries like YOU are? Well, it's because loss of flexibility and aging go hand in hand. But did you know that having good flexibility can slow down aging…no matter how old you are?

These might all just seem like the little nuisances of aging, but unless you begin to actively move your body and increase your joints' range of motion, the degenerating process becomes self-perpetuating. This then further reduces the activities you can do and increases the strain on joints as your body can no longer move freely. Before you realize it, even if you're only in your 40s, 50s, or 60s, you're looking and feeling "old" and not always able to do the things that you would like to do.

Shortened muscles also increase your risk for falling and make it harder to do activities that require flexibility, such as climbing stairs. Warning signs that it's becoming a problem would be having difficulty putting on your shoes and socks or tucking in the back of your shirt.

Not only do you look and feel old, your body is actually aging prematurely!

Fortunately, you don't need to follow this pathway. Even if you are already on it, you can take easy action to begin reversing this trend. I'm here to tell you that you can regain your flexibility no matter how old you are, and by maintaining your flexibility, you can slow down the aging process instead of allowing yourself to have a body that will quickly become stiff, weak, and frail.

Remember, the fitter your body, the younger your cells will be. Strength and flexibility equal a more youthful body!

All it takes is ten minutes a day!

If you are interested in learning more about what you can do to specifically address your flexibility, you can order our *Stretching eBook* pictured here. Go to www.level4pt.com/whgifts to download it.

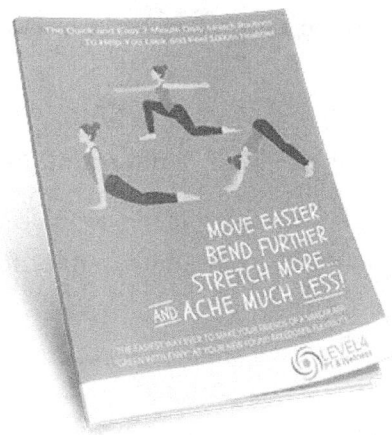

Using Pilates to Increase Flexibility and Reduce Pain

"In 10 sessions you'll feel the difference, in 20 years you'll see the difference, and in 30 you'll have a new body."
– Joseph Pilates

As mentioned in the previous section, as people age, they lose flexibility in their joints and soft tissue. They also experience changes in coordination and balance as well as posture; and let's be honest, a lot of us experience those aches and pains in our hips, our neck, and back.

The reality of being as healthy as you hope to be, staying active for as long as you can, and having your body in good enough condition to let you do all you want to do when you want to do it, is that it does take some effort on your part. There's no getting away from it. I honestly believe that most people know they need to do something to make themselves physically fitter or more active; they're just a bit confused about what the best thing to do is. If that's you, I have a suggestion for you to consider as a top way to reduce the aches and pains associated with growing older: you need to take up Pilates (see Chapter 5 for details on this!).

Another low-impact exercise that I highly recommend—but that many people don't consider to be a serious exercise because of a perceived lack of intensity—is walking.

Six Reasons Walking is the Most Underrated Form of Exercise

Let's dive into what makes walking the most underrated exercise and why you need to make a date with your athletic shoes for a stroll around the block (and beyond!) asap.

1. *Walking is easy.*

It's difficult to motivate yourself to work out knowing there will be soreness later. You don't need an expensive gym membership, classes, or special equipment. All you need is a pair of athletic shoes. Just lace them up, grab your keys, and go—no other gear or planning required. You can literally wear your work clothes and do it on your lunch break. Not to mention, it's free. Everything in life should be so easy.

2. *You can walk (basically) anywhere.*

You can walk in all of the following situations:

- Indoors or outside
- When you travel (It's ideal for sightseeing, though make sure you remember how to get back.)
- At the office (during a phone call or lunchtime)
- Alone or with others
- While shopping!

3. *Walking burns calories.*

Healthy bodies come in all different shapes and sizes, and walking is a wonderful, inclusive exercise for people across the spectrum. Whether you're walking for weight loss, to maintain current weight, or just to keep your other biomarkers in tip-top shape, hitting the treadmill or sidewalk will help you achieve those goals.

If you want to get into the math, walking one mile burns approximately 100 calories; that's not too shabby for 15 to 20 minutes of physical activity. Now if there's a big, fancy dinner on your calendar, get a long walk in beforehand to offset the indulgence, thereby making it guilt-free.

4. *Walking keeps your mind sharp.*

Only one hour of walking for exercise three times a week improves cognition and has the potential to stave off dementia. If you're over the age of 40, what's not to love about a longer attention span and faster problem-solving skills?

5. *Walking helps you live longer.*

Another common theme you've probably noticed throughout this book is that I discuss multiple ways to improve your aging—or how to halt it, rather. When you look at the science, moving—even for just a couple of minutes at a time—strongly influences longevity. It turns out that little things, like taking the stairs in lieu of the elevator, can add up to an increased lifespan. I'll take it!

6. *Walking makes you happy.*

The endorphins would tell you this themselves if they could talk, but walking is a proven mood booster. Just minutes of walking can lead to an upswing in cheerfulness, sociability, and self-confidence.

Ready to give it a try?

Once walking has become routine, another exercise you might want to add to your growing repertoire is strength training.

Strength Training is a Must for Women as They Age

As you get older, you start to lose vitamins and minerals, and health can deteriorate. Your bones become smaller, weaker (osteopenia or osteoporosis), and more prone to serious injuries. You start to lose strength and your cardiovascular health begins its downward spiral. Your skin begins to lose some of its natural elasticity and starts to sag. But it doesn't have to happen quite like this, and strength training can help.

A few of the hundreds of benefits of weightlifting and exercising include the prevention of heart disease, stroke, high blood pressure, diabetes, obesity, back pain, osteoporosis, psychological effects, and many more.

The biggest benefit you might be interested in is how building muscle through strength training increases your metabolism. This is especially important when aging causes hormone levels to shift, which leads to muscle loss and difficulty in losing weight (if that is your goal). Working on increasing your muscle tone by strength training improves your ability to burn fat.

Proper Form is Huge!

This is a big fitness mistake no matter how old you are—poor form when lifting weights and doing exercises can lead to a huge range of injuries—but it's especially important as you age, as joints and muscles deteriorate and become less able to resist damage. I recommend booking regular refresher courses on how to work out safely from a physical therapist instead of from an online personal trainer or a video on YouTube.

Shift Your Workouts

Those bizarre and crazy workouts of your 20s are no good anymore. One-rep maxes and lifting tractor tires like Rocky are still within our capacity, but we pay for them with soreness and injuries.

Instead, focus on medium-weight, medium-rep exercises with large ranges of motion. Good choices that produce exactly the kind of strength and flexibility your body needs include:

- kettlebells
- barbell or dumbbell exercises

Listen to Your Body

If something doesn't feel right or normal, it could be an injury waiting to happen. It's often best for your long-term health to take a moment to evaluate your movement and your pain, determining whether it's a serious threat or simply a part of the everyday discomfort of a workout.

The Importance of a Constantly Varied Exercise Routine

I know you may be thinking that I'm throwing a lot at you by simply saying to *do this* and *do that*. If it were only that easy. I get it. Trust me, I am a physical therapist. Getting people to do exercises is a major challenge in itself. I understand exercising can be tough—and even tougher to sustain. For some people, that's a big enough obstacle to even starting in the first place and a reason why so many people look and feel unhealthy. They don't do much to keep fit because they know they're unlikely to be able to sustain it, so what's the point of starting?

Have you ever felt like that? I know many people who have. And the answer? Well, all you have to do is forget about keeping fit altogether. That's right, forget it! It's not the only way to feel healthier.

Instead, here's what I want you to do: just focus on *being* active. Same thing, you say? Not quite. It's a shift in the way you think and how you see the task at hand, and it will make it more likely that you'll sustain being active for longer. By keeping active, you can get the same health benefits, the ones that are going to keep your joints supple and your heart and lungs in better shape, that a fit person has. The only difference is that being active is easier to sustain. Keeping active can be really fun, for instance, if you take advantage of being able to enjoy the outdoors. And if you enjoy what you're doing, that means you're much more likely to keep doing it.

One of the most important things to take away from this chapter is that if you are considering taking part in any type of increased exercise program (or activity), you must *constantly vary your activity*. Now you have stretching, Pilates, walking, and strength training, and you can add some swimming in there, too.

Mix any of these and you'll dramatically lower your chances of repetitive strain type injuries. I also hope that you will not overlook the secret to success—consistency and hard work.

An important note: Individuals taking part in any form of increased exercise should always check with their primary doctor.

CONCLUSION

LADIES, let's take action!

What You Can Do NOW to Improve Your Health as You Age

If you are experiencing ANY of the issues that you read about so far in this book, I urge you to take these simple steps without delay!

1. *Look up "Pelvic Floor Physical Therapist"* in your area (this is one good way to use Google ☺). Then ask if you can speak to a specialist or do a free consultation to get more information. In all states in the USA no referral from a medical doctor is required. If no one will give you information or allow you to speak to a specialist first, then it is probably not the best facility for you to visit. My office is in northern San Diego, but I see people from all over the globe with virtual consults and am happy to find a resource closer to you if you live outside of the area. Just know that sometimes your doctor will not always recommend this option, and it's likely because they might not truly understand how physical therapists can help you. Seeking out a pelvic floor physical therapist is the most important way to get individualized and specialized care!

2. *Start working on your pelvic floor muscles* and testing your ability to do the following simple exercises of elevator breathing and pelvic floor control (NOTE: if you are experiencing painful sex as described in Chapter 7,

these may not be the right exercises for you, yet. Get assessed first or talk to a pelvic floor physical therapist).

Next, here is a great way to working your pelvic floor in more depth than I explained in Chapter 5.

Elevator breathing and control of pelvic floor

Take it up a level by starting with this exercise rather than by starting with a general Kegel. Imagine your pelvic floor muscles as part of a three-story building with an elevator.

1. Imagine the doors of the elevator closing as you squeeze your pelvic floor muscles, then lift from the vaginal area like an elevator moving up to level one of the building (about 30 percent of your pressure).
2. Hold there.

3. Then imagine the elevator lifting to the second floor by lifting the pelvic floor muscles another 30 percent (or about 60 percent of your total pressure).

4. Hold there for a couple of seconds.

5. Then imagine lifting up the pelvic floor muscles via elevator to the third floor at 100 percent of your full strength, and see if you can hold another two to three seconds.

6. Now relax the pelvic floor down to the ground floor where you started with full relaxation.

7. Repeat five times.

Final Thoughts

I hope you were able to get some clarity by reading this book. Maybe you realized you are not alone and that a resource exists to help guide you in the right direction. If you are a woman who has been told "this happens when you age," you fear surgery or don't agree with the advice given that sounded too invasive, you worry that you will continue to feel discomfort for the next ten years, you don't feel right about taking medications to manage an issue, or you just want to feel stronger and more confident about your body, then this book was written for you!

The reason I took this career path was to help guide women who were falling through gaps in a healthcare system that provides scant information related to common issues that women experience. In this book, I touched on the main topics that elicit the most questions related to women who are nearing or have already passed through menopause, and my biggest hope is that I have helped you find the information you needed that will lead you down the path to improved health and wellness.

I have used the tips in this book on myself and on thousands of clients in person and virtually. So, go back to the chapter that kept your attention the most and read it again; then take action, and use the tips given. If you need guidance or have questions, please visit level4pt.com/womens-health for a variety of helpful resources. Thanks for reading!

BONUS SECTION

The pelvic floor exercises ALL women need to do over 40:

1. Inner thigh/pelvic opening: either position, hold at least a minute, breathe deeply as you stretch.

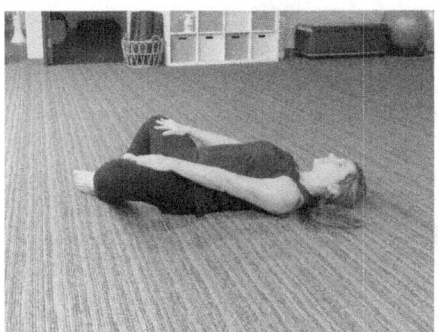
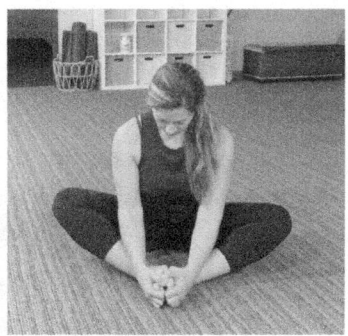

2. Pigeon stretch in elevated position: Hold 1-2 minutes and feel a stretch in the buttock/hip area (the muscles that attach to your tailbone).

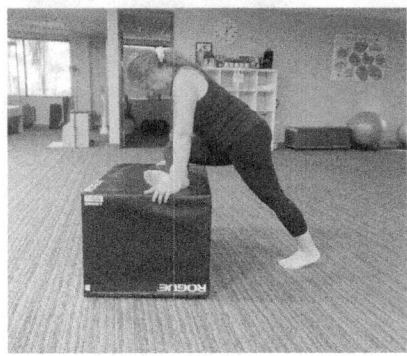

3. Puppy Pose: Think of dropping your navel to the floor and lifting your tailbone up in the air, take 10 deep breaths to release the pelvic floor muscles and upper hamstrings at the pelvic attachment.

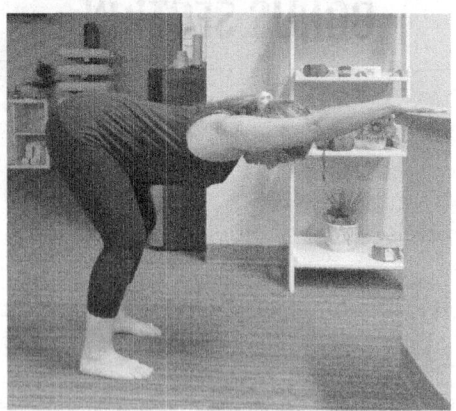

4. Hamstring stretch (with a belt or strap around your foot): Feel a pull in the back of your thigh as you keep the knee straight. Hold 30 sec to one minute, and repeat each side.

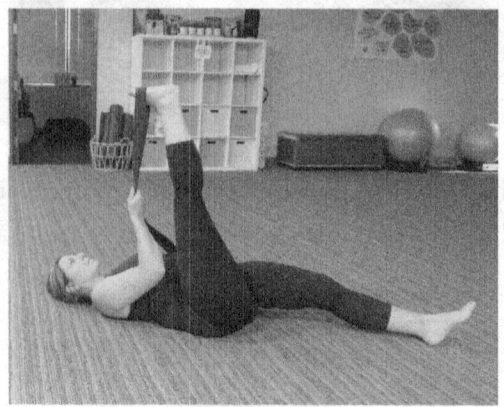

5. Hip flexor stretch: Perform this in front of a couch with a cushion under the knee. Feel a pull in the front of the hip. Hold at least a minute, and tuck your bottom in to get a deeper stretch. Repeat both sides.

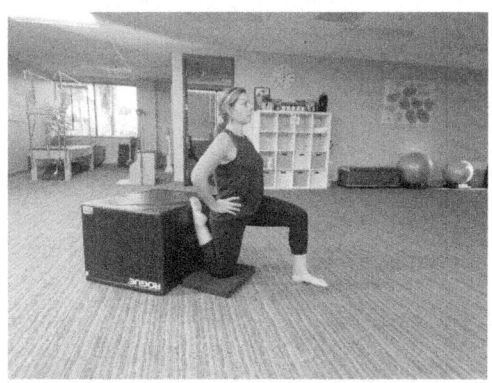

6. Squat to a box/chair behind you. Think of getting your hips back, and keep the chest up. This opens the muscles of your pelvis as you squat and will strengthen the gluteal muscles which stabilize your pelvis externally. Repeat 10 to 15 times, two to three sets a day.

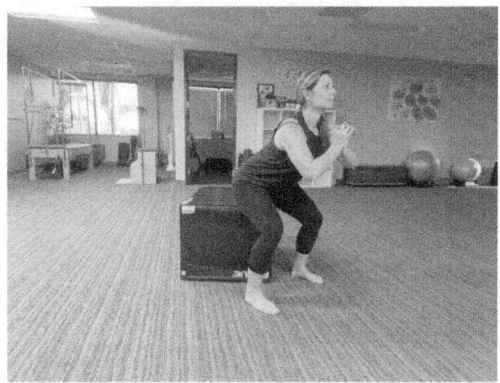

REFERENCES

1. Neels, Hedwig, et al. "Knowledge of the Pelvic Floor in Menopausal Women and in Peripartum Women." *Journal of Physical Therapy Science,* no. 11, Society of Physical Therapy Science, 2016, pp.3020-29. *Crossref,* doi:10.1589/jpts.28.3020.

2. Nygaard, I., et al. "Exercise and Incontinence." *International Journal of Gynecology & Obstetrics,* no 4, Wiley, Dec. 1990, pp. 384-384. *Crossref,* doi: 10.1016/0020-7292(90)90554-x.

3. Gugliotta, Marinella, et al. "Surgical versus Conservative Treatment for Lumbar Disc Herntiation: A Prospective Cohort Study." *BMJ Open,* no. 12, BMJ, Dec. 2016, p.e012938. *Crossref,* doi: 10.1136/bmjopen-2016-012938.

4. Mohan, Yasmina, et al. "Size Matters in Planning Hysterectomy Approach." *Women's Health,* no.4, SAGE Publications, July 2016, pp. 400-03. *Crossref,* doi:10.1177/1745505716653692.

YOUR HEALTH RESOURCE LIBRARY

GET YOUR ADDITIONAL FREE HEALTH AND WELLNESS GUIDES FROM THE LEVEL4 SPECIALISTS NOW.

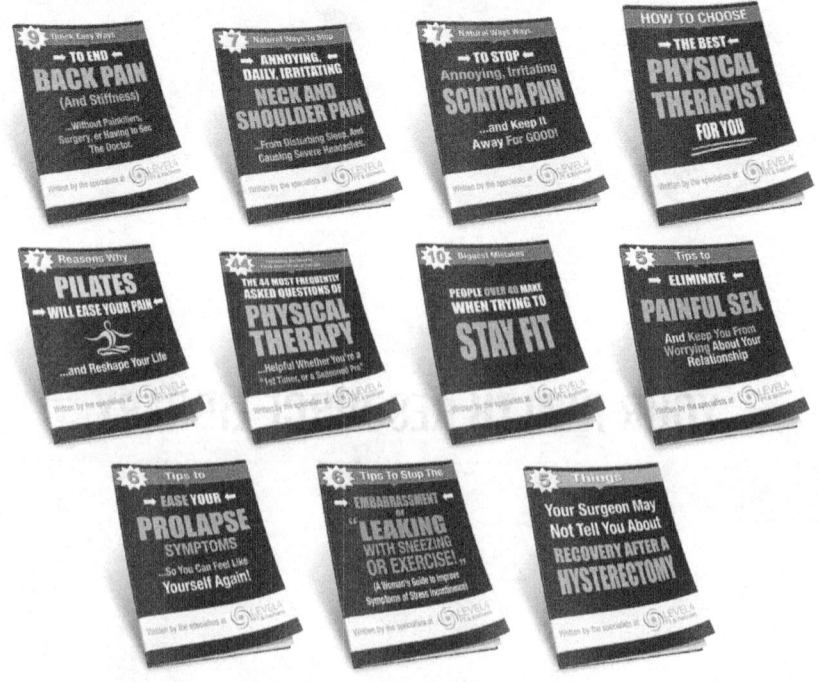

Go to: www.level4pt.com

to get instant access to these amazing free tips guides NOW.

Claim your $300 worth of health and wellness tips that have helped thousands of women become healthier, avoid unnecessary surgeries, and live free from medications…so they can continue living the active lifestyle they want…and deserve. It's absolutely FREE!

Claim your copies now at

www.level4pt.com

HEALTH DISCLAIMER

We make every effort to ensure that we accurately represent the health advice and prognoses displayed throughout this book; however, the information and examples of injuries and their prognoses are based on typical representations of those that we commonly see in our physical therapy clinic. The information given is not intended to apply to every individual's potential injury. As with any issue, each person's symptoms can vary widely, and each person's recovery can also vary depending upon background, genetics, previous medical history, application of exercises, posture, motivation to follow physical therapist advice, and various other physical factors.

It is impossible to give a 100 percent complete accurate diagnosis and prognosis without a thorough physical examination, and likewise, the advice given for management of an injury cannot be deemed fully accurate in the absence of an examination from one of our physical therapists at The Andalon Company, Inc. We are able to offer this service at a standard charge. Significant injury risk is possible if you do not follow due diligence and seek suitable professional advice about your injury. No guarantee of specific results is expressly made or implied in this book.

We do not guarantee the accuracy, completeness, effectiveness, or timeliness of such information. The Information provided is not meant as a substitute for professional advice from a healthcare or other professional. If you act upon this information without consulting with an appropriate professional, you do so at your own risk. It is your responsibility to evaluate text, content, videos, opinions, statements, suggestions, strategies, tactics, or other information available throughout this book. Under no circumstances will The Andalon Company, Inc., or any of our professionals, be liable for any damage caused by reliance on any information we make available.

Made in the USA
Monee, IL
24 April 2025